Andrea Herrmann

Comparison of a global submission of new biological or chemical entity

Andrea Herrmann

Comparison of a global submission of new biological or chemical entity

Strategic decisions and criteria for implementation

Südwestdeutscher Verlag für Hochschulschriften

Impressum/Imprint (nur für Deutschland/only for Germany)
Bibliografische Information der Deutschen Nationalbibliothek: Die Deutsche Nationalbibliothek verzeichnet diese Publikation in der Deutschen Nationalbibliografie; detaillierte bibliografische Daten sind im Internet über http://dnb.d-nb.de abrufbar.
Alle in diesem Buch genannten Marken und Produktnamen unterliegen warenzeichen-, marken- oder patentrechtlichem Schutz bzw. sind Warenzeichen oder eingetragene Warenzeichen der jeweiligen Inhaber. Die Wiedergabe von Marken, Produktnamen, Gebrauchsnamen, Handelsnamen, Warenbezeichnungen u.s.w. in diesem Werk berechtigt auch ohne besondere Kennzeichnung nicht zu der Annahme, dass solche Namen im Sinne der Warenzeichen- und Markenschutzgesetzgebung als frei zu betrachten wären und daher von jedermann benutzt werden dürften.

Verlag: Südwestdeutscher Verlag für Hochschulschriften GmbH & Co. KG
Heinrich-Böcking-Str. 6-8, 66121 Saarbrücken, Deutschland
Telefon +49 681 37 20 271-1, Telefax +49 681 37 20 271-0
Email: info@svh-verlag.de

Approved by: Bonn, Rheinische Friedrich-Wilhelm-Universität, Diss., 2011

Herstellung in Deutschland:
Schaltungsdienst Lange o.H.G., Berlin
Books on Demand GmbH, Norderstedt
Reha GmbH, Saarbrücken
Amazon Distribution GmbH, Leipzig
ISBN: 978-3-8381-3071-2

Imprint (only for USA, GB)
Bibliographic information published by the Deutsche Nationalbibliothek: The Deutsche Nationalbibliothek lists this publication in the Deutsche Nationalbibliografie; detailed bibliographic data are available in the Internet at http://dnb.d-nb.de.
Any brand names and product names mentioned in this book are subject to trademark, brand or patent protection and are trademarks or registered trademarks of their respective holders. The use of brand names, product names, common names, trade names, product descriptions etc. even without a particular marking in this works is in no way to be construed to mean that such names may be regarded as unrestricted in respect of trademark and brand protection legislation and could thus be used by anyone.

Publisher: Südwestdeutscher Verlag für Hochschulschriften GmbH & Co. KG
Heinrich-Böcking-Str. 6-8, 66121 Saarbrücken, Germany
Phone +49 681 37 20 271-1, Fax +49 681 37 20 271-0
Email: info@svh-verlag.de

Printed in the U.S.A.
Printed in the U.K. by (see last page)
ISBN: 978-3-8381-3071-2

Copyright © 2012 by the author and Südwestdeutscher Verlag für Hochschulschriften GmbH & Co. KG and licensors
All rights reserved. Saarbrücken 2012

List of Abbreviations

ACCSQ PPWG	ASEAN Consultative Committee on Standards and Quality Pharmaceutical Product Working Group
ACTD	ASEAN Common Technical Document
ACTR	ASEAN Common Technical Requirements
ADCC	Antibody Dependent Cell-mediated Cytotoxicity
ADEC	Australian Drug Evaluation Committee
ADEPT	Antibody Directed Enzyme Prodrug Therapy
AFR	Africa
AFTA	ASEAN Free Trade Agreement
AIDS	Acquired Immune Deficiency Syndrome
AMG	German Drug Law ("Arzneimittelgesetz")
ANDA	Abbreviated New Drug Application
ANVISA	Brazilian Health Surveillance Agency
API	Active pharmaceutical ingredient
AR	Assessment Report
ASEAN	Association of South-East Asian Nations
ATC	Anatomical Therapeutic Chemical / Defined Daily Dose Classification
AUS	Australia
BLA	Biologics License Application
CA	Competent Authority
CADREAC	Collaboration Agreement of Drug Regulatory Authorities in European Union Associated Countries
CATEME	Câmara Técnica de Medicamentos (the technical board for medicinal products)
CBER	Center for Biologics Evaluation and Research

CCP	Common CADREAC Procedure
CDC	Complement Dependent Cytotoxicity
CDER	Center for Drug Evaluation and Research
CEP	Certificate of suitability
CFR	Code of Federal Regulations
CH	Switzerland
CHMP	The Committee for Medicinal Products for Human Use
CMD	Coordination group for mutual recognition procedures and decentralized procedures – human
CMS	Concerned Member State
CO	Clinical Overview
CoA(s)	Certificate(s) of analysis
COMSI	Coordenação de Medicamentos Sintéticos e Semi-Sintéticos (Synthetic and Semi- Synthetic Medicinal Products Coordination)
CoO	Country of Origin
CP	Centralized Procedure
CPBIH	Coordenação de Productos Biológicos e Hemoterápicos (Hemotherapic and Biologic Medicinal Products Coordination)
CPMP	Committee for Proprietary Medicinal Products
CPP	Certificate of a Pharmaceutical Product
CRF	Case Report Form
CRO	Contract Research Organization
CRT	Case Report Tabulation
CTA	Clinical Trial Application
CTD	Common Technical Document
CV	Curriculum Vitae
DCP	Decentralized Procedure

DMF	Drug Master File
DNA	Deoxyribonucleic acid
DOU	Diário Oficial da Uniao (Brazilian Official Gazette)
DP	Drug Product
DRA	Drug Regulatory Authority
DS	Drug Substance
eCTD	Electronic Common Technical Document
E guidelines	Efficacy ICH guidelines
EC	European Commission
EDMF	European Drug Master File
EDQM	European Directorate for the Quality of Medicines & HealthCare
EE	Eastern Europe
EEA	European Economic Area
EEC	European Economic Community
EGFR	Epidermal Growth Factor Receptor
EMA	European Medicines Agency
EMEA	The European Agency for the Evaluation of Medicinal Products
ErbB	Epidermal growth factor receptor
EU	European Union
FDA	Food and Drug Administration
FDAMA	Food and Drug Administration Modernization Act of 1997
FFDCA	Federal Food, Drug and Cosmetic Act
FIOCRUZ	Fundação Oswaldo Cruz (Oswaldo Cruz Foundation)
FOI	Freedom of Information
GGMED	General office of drugs (Gerência-geral de Medicamentos)
GMP	Good Manufacturing Practice

GPBEN	Coordenação de Pesquisa, Ensayos Clínicos, Medicamentos Biológicos e Nomos (NET Medicinal Products; Biológicas; Research and Clinical Studies Division)
HACA	human anti-chimeric antibodies
HAMA	human anti-mouse antibodies
HER	Human Epidermal growth factor Receptor
HSA	Health Sciences Authority
IgG1	Immunoglobulin G1
ICH	International Conference of Harmonization
INCQS	Instituto National de Controle de Qualidade em Saúde (National institute of quality control and health)
IND	Investigational New Drug Application
INN	International Nonproprietary Names
IP	Intellectual Properties
IRB	Institutional Review Board
ISE	Integrated Summary of Efficacy
ISS	Integrated Summary of Safety
JP	Japan
JPh	Japanese Pharmacopoeia
LA	Latin America
M	Master
M guidelines	Multidisciplinary ICH guidelines
MA	Marketing Authorization
MAA	Marketing Authorization Application
mAb	Monoclonal Antibody
MAC	Medicines Advisory Committee
MAH	Marketing Authorization Holder

MAPP	Manual of Policies and Procedures
MCB	Master Cell Bank
MCRC	Medical Clinical Research Committee
ME	Middle East
MHRA	Medicines and Healthcare products Regulatory Agency
moAb	Monoclonal Antibody
MoH	Ministry of Health
MRA	Mutual Recognition Agreements
MRF	Medicines Registration Form
MR(P)	Mutual Recognition (Procedure)
MS	Member State
n.a.	not applicable
NBE	New Biological Entity
nC	nCADREAC (New Collaboration Agreement between Drug Regulatory Authorities in Central and Eastern European Countries)
nCADREAC	New Collaboration Agreement between Drug Regulatory Authorities in Central and Eastern European Countries
nC-CCC	nCADREAC concerned candidate countries
NCE	New Chemical Entity
NCO	Non Clinical Overview
NDA	New Drug Application
NP	National Procedure
NtA	Notice to Applicants
OTC	Over the Counter
PD	Pharmacodynamic
PDUFA	Prescription Drug User Fee Act

PFS	Progression Free Survival
Ph. Eur.	European Pharmacopoeia
PIL	Patient Information Leaflet/Package Leaflet
PIP	Pediatric Investigational Plan
PK	Pharmacokinetic
PMF	Plasma Master File
PRD	Product Registration Dossier
PRISM	Pharmaceutical Regulatory and Information Systems
PSUR	Period Safety Update Report
QC	Quality Control
Q guidelines	Quality ICH guidelines
QOS	Quality Overall Summary
REN	Renewal
RMS	Reference Member State
RTF	Refusal-To-File
S guidelines	Nonclinical (Safety) ICH guidelines
SCCHN	Squamous Cell Cancer of the Head and Neck
scFv	single-chain Fv fragment
SEA	South East Asia and Western Pacific
SEE	South Eastern Europe
SMF	Site Master File
SOP	Standard Operating Procedure
SOPP	Manual of Standard Operating Procedures and Policies
SPA	Special Protocol Assessment
SPC	Summary of Product Characteristics
SPC	Supplementary Protection Certificate

SUS	Unified Health System
SWOT	Strengths, Weakness, Opportunities and Threats
TGA	Therapeutic Goods Administration
TGFα	transforming growth factor α
ToC(s)	Table of Content(s)
TPD	Therapeutic Products Division
UAR	Update Assessment Report
UK	United Kingdom
UNIAP	Unidade de Atendimento e Protocolo (Services and Filing Unit)
US	United States
USAN	United States Adopted Name
USP	Pharmacopoeia of the United States
USA	United States of America
USR	Urgent Safety Restriction
VAR	Variation
WHO	World Health Organization

Table of Contents

List of Abbreviations		5
Table of Contents		13
List of Appendices		15
Abstract		17
1	Introduction	20
2	Status as of Today	21
3	Analysis of the Pharmaceutical Legislation and Regulatory Requirements for Applying for a Marketing Authorization Application for a New Biological Entity and a New Chemical Entity	26
3.1	ICH	26
3.2	EU	29
3.2.1	Format and content of a Marketing Authorization Application Dossier – Regulatory Requirements	29
3.2.2	Different Marketing Authorization Procedures in EU	30
3.3	USA	38
3.3.1	Dossier Format – ICH CTD	38
3.3.2	Dossier Requirements	38
3.3.3	Registration Procedures	41
3.4	CADREAC	47
3.4.1	General Information	47
3.4.2	Dossier Format – ICH CTD	51
3.4.3	Dossier Requirements	51
3.4.4	Registration Procedures - Example Croatia	56
3.5	ASEAN	64
3.5.1	General Information Regarding ASEAN	64
3.5.2	Dossier Format – ASEAN CTD	66
3.5.3	Dossier Requirements	68
3.5.4	Registration Procedures	70
3.6	CHINA	77
3.6.1	Dossier Format	77
3.6.2	Dossier Requirements	77
3.6.3	Registration Procedures	81
3.7	BRAZIL	83
3.7.1	Dossier Format	83
3.7.2	Dossier Requirements	85
3.7.3	Registration Procedures	86

4	Comparison of the Pharmaceutical Legislation and Regulatory Requirements for a Marketing Authorization Application of a New Biological Entity and a New Chemical Entity within the Different Countries and Regions	93
5	Development of the Global Regulatory Strategy for a New Marketing Authorization Application for a New Compound	115
5.1	Development of a New Compound	115
5.2	Short Introduction of a Monoclonal Antibody	124
5.2.1	Definition	124
5.2.2	Antibody structure	125
5.2.3	Antibody Function	125
5.2.4	Types of Monoclonal Antibodies	126
5.2.5	Goals of Monoclonal Antibodies	127
5.2.6	Cancer Treatment	128
5.2.7	Conclusion Monoclonal Antibodies	129
5.2.8	Manufacturing Process of a New Biotech Product, Example of a Monoclonal Antibody	130
5.3	Development of a Monoclonal Antibody	133
5.3.1	Compound & Mode of Action	134
5.3.2	Development Objectives	134
5.4	Development of the Global Regulatory Strategy for a Monoclonal Antibody	135
5.4.1	Executive Summary of the Regulatory Strategy	135
5.4.2	Regulatory Activities	136
5.4.3	Regional Strategies for Initial Application in ICH	138
5.4.4	Marketing Authorization Strategy for Roll-out to Japan and to non-ICH-countries for the Monoclonal Antibody Monotuximab	139
5.5	Summary and Discussion	145
6	Conclusion and Outlook	154
6.1	Recommendation which Regulatory Procedure to use for which Product	154
6.2	Recommendations for the Development of a Global Regulatory Strategy	155
7	Preliminary Publications and Presentations	161
8	Appendices	162
9	Bibliography	259

List of Appendices

APPENDIX 1	CTD TABLE OF CONTENTS	162
APPENDIX 2	CTD TABLE OF CONTENT FOR EU MODULE 1	167
APPENDIX 3	DIFFERENCES NBE AND NCE WITH REGARD TO MODULE 2 AND 3	168
APPENDIX 4	TABLE OF CONTENTS FOR AN NDA IN USA	178
APPENDIX 5	TABLE OF COMPARISON OF MECHANISMS TO HASTEN PRODUCT AVAILABILITY IN USA	183
APPENDIX 6	TABLE OF SPECIFIC NATIONAL REQUIREMENTS OF NCADREAC DRAS CONCERNED	184
APPENDIX 7	INFORMATION SHARING LETTER	196
APPENDIX 8	REPORT ON THE REPORT ON THE MARKETING AUTHORISATION GRANTED BY THE NCADREAC DRA CONCERNED OF THE MEDICINAL PRODUCT SUBJECTED TO THE MUTUAL RECOGNITION PROCEDURE IN THE EU	197
APPENDIX 9	TABLE OF CONTENTS FOR ACTD	198
APPENDIX 10	DOSSIER REQUIREMENTS FOR QUALITY PART OF THE DOSSIER FOR ASEAN COUNTRIES	200
APPENDIX 11	DOSSIER REQUIREMENTS FOR AN NCE IN CHINA	206
APPENDIX 12	TABLE OF APPLICATION INFORMATION ITEM FOR CHINA	208
APPENDIX 13	DOSSIER REQUIREMENTS FOR AN NBE IN CHINA	210
APPENDIX 14	TABLE OF APPLICATION INFORMATION ITEMS FOR CHINA	213
APPENDIX 15	ADMINISTRATIVE DOCUMENTS ARE REQUIRED FOR NEW MEDICINAL PRODUCTS WHICH ARE IMPORTED TO BRAZIL	218
APPENDIX 16	DOSSIER REQUIREMENTS (PHARMACEUTICAL/ CHEMICAL/ BIOLOGICAL, PRECLINICAL AND CLINICAL DOCUMENTATION) FOR BRAZIL	220
APPENDIX 17	ROUTE MAP FOR CREATION OF A CTD DOSSIER FOR MAA	226
APPENDIX 18	AN EXAMPLE FOR A GLOBAL PLAN:	241
APPENDIX 19	AVAILABLE GUIDELINES AND REGULATIONS	244
APPENDIX 20	SUMMARY TABLE CONCERNING THE REGULATORY STRATEGY FOR THE MA FOR THE DIFFERENT COUNTRIES	250
APPENDIX 21	REQUIREMENTS TABLES	252

Abstract

The world covers more than 190 countries in which at the moment in most of them pharmaceutical legislations and regulatory requirements are established and implemented, e.g. to describe the marketing authorization (MA) procedure for medicinal products.
To be able to submit a marketing authorization application (MAA) in all these countries, it is important to know exactly the pharmaceutical legislations (regulations, directives and guidelines) and the regulatory requirements in each of the country in advance.
The objective of the pharmaceutical companies is to identify ways and factors that impede the efficient registration of new medicinal products and their timely access to patients. Due to the fact that the European Union (EU) and the United States (US) are the biggest and most potential markets for medicinal products in the world, global working companies focus and analyze the EU and US pharmaceutical legislations and regulatory requirements very detailed in advance and include these requirements from EU and US normally in their development concept of a new medicinal product and consequently in their global regulatory strategy for MAA of this product. But the industry recognized in the last few years also that the other regions of the world – Japan (JP), Latin America (LA), Middle East (ME)/Africa (AFR) and South East Asia (SEA), and are becoming increasingly important to pharmaceutical companies in their global marketing strategies. Therefore companies with global approach realize that it is not sufficient anymore to develop their global regulatory strategy based on the regulatory requirements in EU and US but also to take into consideration the other regions of the world.

Therefore within this dissertation a scientific evaluation and recommendation for the development of a new compound (new biological entity (NBE) or new chemical entity (NCE)) is provided. Based on these recommendations for a global development for a new compound, a regulatory strategy for an NBE on the example of a monoclonal antibody (mAb) is provided.

First, the different pharmaceutical legislations and regulatory requirements for a new MAA of an NBE and NCE based on the examples of EU, United States of America (USA), Collaboration Agreement of Drug Regulatory Authorities in European Union Associated Countries (CADREAC) (example: Croatia), LA (Brazil) and SEA ((Association of South-East Asian Nations (ASEAN): example Singapore) and China) are discussed and analyzed in detail. The analyses are made especially concerning the aspects required and accepted dossier format, dossier requirements (documents required for an MAA) and different regulatory procedures for MAAs. Also the aspects concerning confidentiality of the documentation submitted to the different authorities, the IP (intellectual property) rights and patent issues are covered shortly.

Afterwards the comparison between the different pharmaceutical and regulatory legislations in these countries and the comparison between MAAs for NBEs and NCEs follows.

Based on this comparison the general aspects of a global development for a new compound (NBE or NCE) are discussed. The differences in global development between an NBE and an NCE are also covered within this dissertation. Based on this general strategy for global development of new compounds a global regulatory strategy for an NBE on the example of a mAb is developed.

As the pharmaceutical legislations and requirements are permanently changing it is of utmost importance that pharmaceutical companies check the current legislations and requirements before starting a global development of a new compound. Also during the development of a new compound the changes in pharmaceutical legislations and regulations have to be checked and have to be incorporated in the global strategy in order to submit a MA dossier according to current requirements. This will ensure that the authorities accept the MA because of following regulations or guidelines. In case a regulation or guideline is not followed the applicant has to be present a justification for doing this approach and it cannot be guaranteed that authorities will accept this. Therefore it is strongly recommended to check the requirements and fulfill all requirements to be able to get an approval for the MA dossier of the newly developed compound.

The requirements to get a medicinal product approved increase constantly and it can be anticipated that they will increase further. During the last years the tendency can be observed that more patient tailored drugs are requested by authorities compared to products approved in very broad indications. This might be not so beneficial from a company perspective as the number of patients which can be treated with one medicinal product which is patient tailored might be smaller. Nevertheless, this is the direction agencies might follow in future. Therefore topics like biomarkers or other specific markers to identify patient tailored drugs will become more and more of importance in future. It is advisable for companies to include biomarkers or other specific markers in their development program of a new compound as otherwise authorities might not grant the submitted MA.

In addition to the increasing requirements by authorities to get a new medicinal product registered, the pharmaceutical environment will change due to greater influences of governments and changing health care systems. It has to be awaited how governments will build up the health care systems in future and how requirements will change. It is most likely that the prices for new medicines will be limited by governments to relieve the health care systems and that requirements to get medicinal products reimbursed will also increase in future. Studies to proof a positive cost benefit ratio might be required for each new medicinal product as a prerequisite to get the product reimbursed.

In conclusion the requirements to get a drug registered and reimbursed will increase and consequently the development costs for companies will increase, too.

One possible solution to deal with the increased costs for development and the increasing requirements might be that pharmaceutical companies will merge and will develop new innovative medicinal products together and share the development costs. This will be especially attractive for small and medium-sized companies. Also companies might think about the location of their development centers in order optimize the development. It is recommended that companies will have only one or two global development centers where the global development for all new compounds is done.

Pharmaceutical companies should be in closed contact with authorities in order to be able to fulfill all requirements needed to get a new medicinal product approved and marketed. Companies should be also in close contacts with governments especially regarding health care systems in order to fulfill their requirements and in order to be able to influence them with regard to decisions on health care systems.

Besides all increasing barriers for getting new products approved and marketed, it is of utmost importance that the development of new innovative medicinal products will be continued to offer patients best medicinal supply.

Therefore it seems to be logical that pharmaceutical companies, authorities and governments have to work together and find solutions that the development of new innovative drugs will be attractive and efficient for all sites in future.

1 Introduction

Today, the regulatory requirements in the various countries of the world are still quite different. Therefore it is very difficult - especially for companies with global activities - to develop one single regulatory approach for a marketing authorization application (MAA) for a new medicinal product on the basis of one dossier submitted simultaneously to various countries in the world.

On this background it is very important to know in detail the regulatory requirements in each concerned country where an MAA should be submitted to establish a suitable regulatory strategy before the submission in order to avoid any major difficulties and unexpected surprises.

The dissertation topic "Comparison of a global submission of new biological entity and a new chemical entity – strategic decisions and criteria for implementation" as a first focus includes the development of a global regulatory strategy for the submission of an MAA of a new compound (new biological entity (NBE) or new chemical entity (NCE)). For this strategy which is based on my personal professional experiences in pharmaceutical industry a detailed analysis of the pharmaceutical legislations and regulatory requirements in the different regions (International Conference of Harmonization (ICH) countries (which are European Union (EU), Japan (JP) and United States of America (USA)) and non-ICH-countries) and countries over the world is made. The analysis is focused especially to identify and discuss the commonness and the main differences. Based on the result of the analysis of the pharmaceutical legislation and regulatory requirements for NBEs and NCEs worldwide, a general strategy for the development of a new compound (NBE or NCE) is provided. The general strategy for the development of a new compound results then into the development of a global regulatory strategy for the submission of a new MAA of an NBE on the example of a monoclonal antibody (mAb).

2 Status as of Today

The United Nations cover 192 countries in which at the moment in most of them pharmaceutical legislations and regulatory requirements are established and implemented, e.g. to describe the marketing authorization (MA) procedure for medicinal products.

To be able to submit an MAA in all the major markets, it is important to know exactly the pharmaceutical legislations (regulations, directives, and guidelines) and the regulatory requirements in each of the country in advance. Differences in the pharmaceutical legislations and regulatory requirements can be found for example in the requirement for administrative data (e.g. type of documents which are requested, legalization necessary, etc.), in the pharmaceutical data (e.g. in the requirements for stability data (ICH versus ASEAN) and also in the clinical data (e.g. placebo-controlled studies or comparative studies). Therefore, it is very important to analyze and discuss especially the differences and commonness between the pharmaceutical legislations and regulatory requirements in the different countries of the world.

Due to the fact that the EU and United States (US) are the biggest and most potential markets for medicinal products in the world, globally working companies focus and analyze the EU and US pharmaceutical legislations and regulatory requirements very detailed in advance and include these requirements from EU and US normally in their development concept of a new medicinal product and consequently in their global regulatory strategy for the MAA of this product.

In the last few years pharmaceutical companies recognized that other regions of the world –Japan (JP), Latin America (LA), South Eastern Europe (SEE), Middle East/Africa (ME/AFR) and South East Asia and Western Pacific (SEA), and are becoming increasingly important for pharmaceutical companies in their global marketing strategies. The objective of the companies is to identify ways and factors that impede the efficient registration of new medicinal products and their timely access to patients.

Therefore companies with global approach realize that it is not sufficient anymore to develop their global regulatory strategy based on the regulatory requirements in EU and US but also to take into consideration the other regions of the world.

Consequently, a detailed analysis of the pharmaceutical legislations and regulatory requirements in Eastern Europe (EE), LA and SEA are necessary - in addition to the detailed analysis of the pharmaceutical legislations and regulatory requirements in EU and USA - to be finally able to develop a global regulatory strategy for an MAA of a new compound (NBE or NCE). The third country of ICH – JP - is not covered by this thesis.

The pharmaceutical legislations and regulatory requirements in the world were established during the last 100 years, often as results of some tragedies. 1937, in the USA 100 people died after consumption of a children's syrup (Diethylene glycol poisoning) and based on this in 1938 the first Food Drug and Cosmetic Act was implemented. The resulting Food Drug and Cosmetic Act of 1938 required that proof, in the form of a New Drug Application (commonly called an NDA) has to be submitted to a new department called the US Food and Drug Administration (FDA). Anyone wishing to market a "New Drug" has to show safety for intended use in the form of an NDA.

In Germany, the first Drug Law was established in 1961 and was implemented soon afterwards the thalidomide tragedy in Europe, which happened in the early sixties. Also in Japan the first drug law was established in 1961. In EU the first drug law was established in 1965 with the Directive 65/65.

The aim of all the regulatory legislations (drug laws) and all drug regulatory authorities (DRAs) is to provide patients with safe medicinal products as fast as possible based on the proof of quality, safety and efficacy which has to be shown by a submission of an MAA.

The changing regulatory requirement and legislations have an impact on the regulatory strategy during drug development.

Consequently, due to the fact that the pharmaceutical legislation in EU was changed some years ago accordingly to the "EU Review 2004", a detailed analysis of the changes in the pharmaceutical legislations and regulatory requirements in EU due to the new EU legislation is necessary, especially the changes concerning the different regulatory procedures and requirements in EU which have an impact on the regulatory strategy.

The changes in the EU legislation have also an impact on other countries in the world which implemented the EU legislations like Serbia or the Collaboration Agreement of Drug Regulatory Authorities in European Union Associated Countries (CADREAC) which are currently only Croatia because most of its regulation depend on EU legislation. CADREAC was renamed to new CADREAC (nCADREAC) after the EU accession of nine of the original CADREAC countries in 2004.

As a result of the review 2004 several regulations and directives have been changed and replaced.

The Council Regulation 2309/93[1] describes the centralized procedure (CP) in the EU and it also has established the European Medicines Agency (EMA) (formerly: The European Agency for the Evaluation of Medicinal Products (EMEA)) (also called "Agency")) and the Committee for Medicinal Products for Human Use (CHMP) (formerly: Committee for Proprietary Medicinal Products ((CPMP)), the scientific committee - which is responsible for the evaluation of new MAAs for medicinal products for human use - under the direction of the Agency.

Due to the review 2004, the Council Regulation 2309/93[1] was replaced by the new Council Regulation 726/2004[2]. This new regulation was adopted on 31st March 2004 and became valid on the 20th May 2004. Other parts of the regulation had to be implemented until 20th November 2005.

After the full implementation of the revised community legislation in November 2005 several changes was made with regard to the CP. These include an expansion of the scope of the procedure, establishment of a procedure for conditional MAs, formalization of an accelerated procedure and management of compassionate use programs. In addition, assistance will be available for small and medium-sized enterprises.

Next to the Council Regulation 2309/93[1] also the directive 2001/83[3] - the codification directive - was amended by Directive 2004/27[4] and 2004/24 (for herbal drugs)[5]. The two Directives 2004/27 and 2004/24 were adopted on 31st March 2004 and had to be implemented into national law. Therefore a transition period of 18 months was foreseen. This meant that the directives had to be implemented into national law of the EU member states (MSs) until November 2005.

---

[1] *Official Journal L 214, 24.08.1993 - Council Regulation (EEC) No 2309/93 of 22 July 1993 laying down Community procedures for the authorisation and supervision of medicinal products for human and veterinary use and establishing a European Agency for the Evaluation of Medicinal Products – page 1 - 211*

[2] *Official Journal L 136, 30.04.2004 - Regulation (EC) No 726/2004 of the European Parliament and of the Council of 31 March 2004 laying down Community procedures for the authorisation and supervision of medicinal products for human and veterinary use and establishing a European Medicines Agency – page 1 ff.*

[3] *Official Journal L 311, 28.11.2001 - Directive 2001/83/EEC of the European Parliament and of the Council of 6 November 2001 on the Community code relating to medicinal products for human use – page 67 – 128*

[4] *Official Journal L 136, 30.04.2004 - Directive 2004/27 EEC of the European Parliament and of the Council of 31 March 2004 amending Directive 2001/83/EC on the Community code relating to medicinal products for human use – page 34 - 57*

[5] *Official Journal L 136, 30.04.2004 - Directive 2004/24/EC of the European Parliament and of the Council of 31 March 2004 amending, as regards traditional herbal medicinal products, Directive 2001/83/EC on the Community code relating to medicinal products for human use – page 85 - 90*

The changes in the EU legislation had also a big impact on the CADREAC countries and their legislations ([6,7]) because the so-called CADREAC procedures are directly linked with the EU legislations and depend on the EU legislation and the EU regulatory procedures.

Another important factor which should be mentioned and discussed in detail is the Association of Southern Asian Nations (ASEAN)[8]. ASEAN was established on 8 August 1967 in Bangkok by the five original member countries Indonesia, Malaysia, Philippines, Singapore and Thailand. On 8 January 1984 Brunei Darussalam joined ASEAN, Vietnam on 28 July 1995, Laos and Myanmar on 23 July 1997, and Cambodia on 30 April 1999.

In 1999 a harmonization initiative was started among the 10 ASEAN countries. One aim of this harmonization should be to harmonize quality guidelines that are valid for all countries involved. Another focus lies in the technical co-operation. Therefore the ASEAN Consultative Committee on Standards and Quality Pharmaceutical Product Working Group (ACCSQ PPWG) was established. The objective of the ACCSQ PPWG is the development of *"harmonization schemes of pharmaceuticals' regulations of the ASEAN member countries to complement and facilitate the objective of ASEAN Free Trade Area (AFTA), particularly, the elimination of technical barriers to trade posed by these regulations, without compromising on drug quality, safety and efficacy."* [8]

ASEAN established the so called ASEAN Common Technical Document (ACTD) and the ASEAN Common Technical Requirements (ACTR) to create harmonized requirements and a common format for all submissions of dossiers in the ASEAN countries. The ACTD is a common format and content acceptable for an application in the ASEAN member countries. The ACTR are a set of written requirements or guidelines intended to provide guidance to applicants in order to be able to prepare application dossiers in a way that is consistent with the expectations of all ASEAN DRAs. [8]

The full implementation of the ASEAN requirements (like ACTD and ACTR) in the ASEAN countries is not yet finalized, a prolongation/transition period is possible. There is an interim period agreed wherein ACTD and national formats allowed in most of the ASEAN countries, whereas in some countries like Singapore ICH CTD is accepted.

---

[6] *Procedure on the granting of marketing authorisations by CADREAC Drug Regulatory Authorities for medicinal products for human use already authorized in the EU following the centralized procedure and the variation and renewal of such marketing authorisations (5th revision of December 21,2001)*

[7] *Procedure on the granting of marketing authorisations by CADREAC Drug Regulatory Authorities for medicinal products for human use already authorized in EU member states following the decentralized procedure (1st revision of June 10,2001)*

[8] *Homepage of ASEAN (Association of Southeast Asian Nationals http://www.aseansec.org/ - dated 27.04.2009*

The full implementation of ACTD for new products was expected by 31 December 2008 whereas the full implementation for currently registered products is expected to be done until 01 January 2012. According to information received from the ASEAN countries (January 2009) some of the ASEAN countries still accept the CTD-format for MAAs of NCEs and NBEs whereas for renewals (RENs) and variations (VARs) only the ACTD-format is accepted by ASEAN countries.

As mentioned before, it is important to know exactly the pharmaceutical legislations (regulations, directives and guidelines) and the regulatory requirements in each of the countries in advance to be able to submit an MAA in all these countries. Based on the result of the analyzes of the pharmaceutical legislation and regulatory requirements for NCEs and NBEs worldwide, a global regulatory strategy for submission of a new MAA of a new compound (NBE or NCE) can be developed and established before the submission in order to avoid any major difficulties and unexpected surprises.

3 Analysis of the Pharmaceutical Legislation and Regulatory Requirements for Applying for a Marketing Authorization Application for a New Biological Entity and a New Chemical Entity

3.1 ICH

The "International Conference on Harmonization of Technical Requirements for the Registration of Pharmaceuticals for Human Use" (ICH) consists of six parties, which represents the regulatory bodies and research-based industry in the three main regions - EU, JP and the USA[9].

ICH was established in 1990 as a joint regulatory authorities/industry project. The purpose of this "institution" is to improve the efficiency of the process for developing and registering new medicinal products in Europe, Japan and the US because in these regions the majority of new medicines are currently developed. This improvement should be achieved through harmonization in order to make these products available to patients with a minimum of delay[9]. Therefore ICH has developed over 50 guidelines with harmonized requirements in order to ensure that the development of medicinal products should be done in the most efficient and cost effective way. In addition the harmonized requirements should minimize the use of animal testing without compromising safety and efficacy and should avoid unneeded duplication of clinical trials in humans.

During the Fifth International Conference on Harmonization (ICH 5) which took place in San Diego in November 2000 the final harmonized Common Technical Document (CTD) was released. The Conference followed the recommendations of the ICH Steering Committee and Expert Working Groups, which took place some days before the conference and wherein the final harmonized Common Technical Document (CTD) was completed.[9]

---

[9] Homepage of ICH (International Conference of Harmonization:
The Fifth International Conference on Harmonization - ICH5 and Steering Committee Meeting
"The Common Technical Document Released Putting It All Together
A Decade of Harmonization" http://www.ich.org/cache/html/454-272-1.html - dated 27.04.2009

The CTD consists of five modules (please refer to attached pyramid). The structure of Module 2, 3, 4 and 5 is common for all ICH regions (EU, JP and USA). The Module 1 is not part of the CTD format and is special for each of the ICH regions.[10]

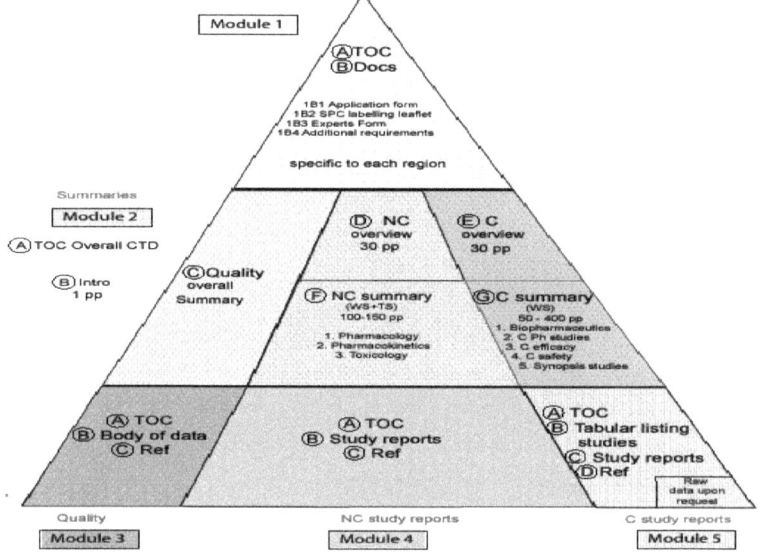

The table of contents (ToCs) of Module 2 – 5 of the ICH CTD dossier is enclosed as an attachment (see "APPENDIX 1: CTD table of contents")[11].

---

[10] *Volume 2B Notice to Applicants (NtA): Medicinal products for human use - Presentation and format of the dossier Common Technical Document (CTD)*
http://ec.europa.eu/enterprise/pharmaceuticals/eudralex/vol2_en.htm#2b
http://ec.europa.eu/enterprise/pharmaceuticals/eudralex/vol-2/b/update_200805/ctd_05-2008.pdf - dated 27.04.2009
[11] http://en.wikipedia.org/wiki/File:CTD_Pyramid.jpg

Modular Structure of Common Technical Document

```
                    Module 1
                    Administrative
                    and prescribing
                    information
                    (not harmonized)

                    Module 2
         ─────────────────────────────────
                Nonclinical    Clinical
        Quality overview       overview
        overall ─────────────────────────
        summary Nonclinical    Clinical
                summary        summary
         ─────────────────────────────────
         Module 3   Module 4    Module 5
         Quality    Nonclinical Clinical
         data       study reports study reports
```

In addition to the CTD format meanwhile the electronic CTD (eCTD) format was established. The eCTD is based on the CTD format and is an interface for pharmaceutical companies to transfer regulatory information to DRAs. The dossiers will be submitted electronically in CTD format to the authorities. Compared to CTD-dossier the Module 1 is part of the eCTD dossier. The eCTD was developed by the ICH Multidisciplinary Group 2 Expert Working Group.[9]

All countries which do not belong to ICH (EU, JP and USA) are covered by the so-called non-ICH-countries. The non-ICH-countries (in total more than 100 countries) have no obligation to establish the ICH-format, nevertheless, some of these countries like Australia (AUS), Canada and Switzerland (CH) established the ICH-format.

To sum up, the CTD is only a common format for the preparation of dossiers for submission to the regulatory authorities in the three ICH regions of EU, JP and USA and gives no information about the content of the dossier. It does not indicate which studies and data are required and should be submitted in order to get an approval. The content of a MAA dossier is described in the corresponding ICH guidelines (Quality (Q) guidelines, Safety (S) guidelines and E (Efficacy guidelines)) and should be identical for all three ICH regions. Nevertheless, it might happen that the dossier is not necessarily completely identical for all regions, because regional requirements may affect the content of the dossier submitted in each region (mainly in the regional section (3.2.R)).[12]

---

[12] *VOLUME 2A NtA - Procedures for marketing authorisation CHAPTER 1 Marketing authorisation from November 2005 http://ec.europa.eu/enterprise/pharmaceuticals/eudralex/vol-2/a/vol2a_chap1_2005-11.pdf - dated 27.04.2009*

The detailed dossier requirements for the ICH regions EU and USA will be described in detail in the chapters for EU (chapter 3.2) and USA (chapter 3.3). As mentioned before the third country of ICH – JP - is not covered by this thesis.

3.2 EU

3.2.1 Format and content of a Marketing Authorization Application Dossier – Regulatory Requirements

In the EU, the regulatory requirements for getting the approval of an MAA are described in the Notice to Applicants (NtA) Volume 2B: "Medicinal products for human use - Presentation and format of the dossier Common Technical Document (CTD)"[10]:
"The CTD gives no information about the content of a dossier and does not indicate which studies and data are required for a successful approval. Regional requirements may affect the content of the dossier submitted in each region, therefore the dossier will not necessarily be identical for all regions.
The CTD indicates an appropriate format for the data that have been required in an application. Applicants should not modify the overall organisation of the Common Technical Document as outlined in the guideline. However, in the Non-clinical and Clinical Summaries, applicants can modify individual formats if needed to provide the best possible tabulated presentation of the technical information, in order to facilitate the understanding and NtA, Vol. 2B-CTD, foreword & introduction, edition June 2006 Page 4 evaluation of the results. The new EU-CTD-presentation will be applicable for all types of marketing authorisation applications irrespective of the procedure (CP, MRP, DCP or national) and of type of application (stand alone, generics etc). The CTD-format will be applicable for all types of products (new chemical entities, radiopharmaceuticals, vaccines, herbals etc.) To determine the applicability of this format for a particular type of product, applicants should consult with the appropriate regulatory authorities."[10]

The CTD dossier is structured in 5 Modules, whereas Module 2, 3, 4 and 5 are part of the CTD.

For the EU the content of the Module 1 is defined in Volume 2B, NtA, Medicinal products for human use, Presentation and format of the dossier- Common Technical Document (CTD): *"The content of Module 1 for EU was defined by the European Commission in consultation with the competent authorities of the Member States, the European Agency for the Evaluation of Medicinal Products and interested parties."*[10]

The Module 1 in the EU consists of the different documents which are listed in appendix 2 ("APPENDIX 2 CTD table of content for EU Module 1")[10].

In summary the CTD is only a common format for the preparation of dossiers for submission to the regulatory authorities in the three ICH regions of EU, JP and USA and gives no information about the content of the dossier. It does not indicate which studies and data are required and should be submitted in order to get an approval. The content of a MAA dossier is described in the corresponding ICH guidelines (Quality (Q) guidelines, Safety (S) guidelines and E (Efficacy guidelines)) and should be identical for all three ICH regions. Nevertheless, it might happen that the dossier is not necessarily identical for all regions, because regional requirements may affect the content of the dossier submitted in each region.[12]

3.2.2 Different Marketing Authorization Procedures in EU

In the EU, there are today four possible registration procedures in order to receive an MAA for a medicinal product: the national procedure, the Decentralized procedure (DCP), the Mutual Recognition Procedure (MRP) and the CP. Depending on the type of the medicinal product, the applicant may have no choice between the procedures and is obliged to use the CP. According to annex of the Regulation 726/2004[2] the CP is mandatory for the following types of medicinal products:

"1. Medicinal products developed by means of one of the following biotechnological processes:

- recombinant Deoxyribonucleic Acid technology,

  - *controlled expression of genes coding for biologically active proteins in prokaryotes and eukaryotes including transformed mammalian cells,*

- *hybridoma and monoclonal methods.*

2. Medicinal products for veterinary use intended primarily for use as performance enhancers in order to promote the growth of treated animals or to increase yields from treated animals.

3. Medicinal products for human use containing a new active substance which, on the date of entry into force of this Regulation, was not authorised in the Community, for which the therapeutic indication is the treatment of any of the following diseases:

- acquired immune deficiency syndrome,
- cancer,
- neurodegenerative disorder
- diabetes

and with effect from 20 May 2008

- *auto-immune diseases and other immune dysfunctions,*
- *viral diseases.*

After 20 May 2008, the Commission, having consulted the Agency, may present any appropriate proposal modifying this point and the Council shall take a decision on that proposal by qualified majority.

4. Medicinal products that are designated as orphan medicinal products pursuant to Regulation (EC) No 141/2000."

In addition the CP is compulsory for advanced therapy medicinal products under the auspices of Regulation (EC) No 1394/2007 (applied from 30-Dec-2008).

The CP is optional for getting the MAs for medicinal products referred to in Article 3(2) of Regulation (EC) No 726/2004: *"relating to medicinal products containing new active substances, products which constitute a significant therapeutic, scientific or technical innovation or products for which the granting of a Community authorisation would be in the interest of patients or animal health at Community level. The applicant has to request confirmation that the product is eligible for evaluation through the centralised procedure (optional scope) and the EMEA will decide on the matter; and a generic medicinal product of a centrally authorised medicinal product if not using the option in Article 3(3) of Regulation (EC) No 726/2004."*[12]

The CP is an option for generics and in the future for MAAs which include data to support the use of the medicinal product in the pediatric population.

The detailed activities and timetables for the different EU procedures (national procedure, CP, MRP and DCP) are not presented within this dissertation, only general aspects regarding the procedures are mentioned.

Besides the normal registration procedures in EU (national procedure, CP, MRP and DCP) there are also some special procedures like Orphan Drug Designation or accelerated assessment procedures. The Orphan Drug Designation is applicable for medicinal product with orphan drug status and is not described here in more details.

Accelerated assessment procedure

In article 33 of Regulation (EC) 726/2004[2] it is mentioned that *"in order to meet, in particular the legitimate expectations of patients and to take account of the increasingly rapid progress of science and therapies, accelerated assessment procedures should be set up, reserved for medicinal products of major therapeutic interest, and procedures for obtaining temporary authorisations subject to certain annually reviewable conditions".*

Therefore accelerated assessment procedure can be used for MAAs of medicinal products which are of major interest from the viewpoint of public health and in particular from the point of view of therapeutic innovation. The applicant can request an accelerated assessment procedure and this request shall be duly well-grounded.[13]

Within the request for an accelerated assessment procedure a justification should be provided that the medicinal product is expected to be of major public health interest particularly from the point of view of therapeutic innovation.[13]

The request for accelerated assessment procedure is submitted to the CHMP. Based on the justification of the applicant and the recommendation of the Rapporteur, the CHMP will make a decision on the request for accelerated assessment. This decision has no influence on the MAA submission. In case the CHMP accepts the request, the time limit for the evaluation of the dossier of 210 days to give an opinion shall be reduced to 150 days.

It is possible that after a request for accelerated assessment procedure has been granted, at any time during the MAA, the CHMP may decide to continue the assessment under standard CP timelines according to Article 6 (3) of Regulation (EC) 726/2004[2]. This might happen in case the CHMP is the opinion that it is no longer appropriate to conduct an accelerated assessment.[13]

The accelerated assessment procedure is not described here in more details.

3.2.2.1 National Procedure

The national procedure for applying for a MA in EU is today only possible if the medicinal product is not yet registered in any other EU MS and if the medicinal product does not fall under Regulation 726/2004[2] for which the CP is mandatory and if a MA is only planned for one MS. In such a case it is possible to apply for a MA via national procedure in one specific MS. The MAA has to follow the national regulations and should be submitted directly to the DRA of this specific MS for evaluation. This national DRA will evaluate the dossier and will grant the national MA in case the evaluation of the dossier is positive. As soon as the medicinal product should then (after approval in the 1st MS) be registered in a 2nd MS the MR procedure has to be used.

In summary today it is not possible any more to register a product in more than one EU member state via national procedure. If the product is intended to be registered in more than one EU MS and the CP is not mandatory the applicant can choose between MRP and DCP.

---

[13] *Guideline on the procedure for accelerated assessment pursuant to articlie 14(9) of regulation (EC) No 726/2004*
http://www.emea.europa.eu/docs/en_GB/document_library/Regulatory_and_procedural_guideli ne/2009/10/WC500004136.pdf - dated 27.04.2009)

3.2.2.2 Centralized Procedure

As mentioned above the Regulation 726/2004[2] and especially the annex of the regulation clearly define which types of medicinal products have obligatorily to use the CP. The CP is mandatory for new active substances for certain therapeutic areas like acquired immune deficiency syndrome (AIDS), cancer or viral diseases and for medicinal products derived from biotechnology. The CP is optional for other innovative new medicinal products (e.g. for medicinal product containing a new active substance, which was not authorized in the EU at the date when the Regulation 726/2004 came into force and for medicinal product for which a significant therapeutic, scientific or technical innovation can be demonstrated). The MAAs have to be submitted directly to the EMA in London.

The scientific evaluation of the MAA submitted to EMA is handled by the CHMP within 210 days. Normally the CHMP gives the assessment of the MAA dossier to two CHMP members of two MS, the so-called "Rapporteur" and "Co-Rapporteur".

The "Rapporteur and Co-Rapporteur" are members of the CHMP who co-ordinate the evaluation of the MAAs. It is possible that the applicant of the MAA indicates in the letter of intent - which has to be submitted to announce the intention of an MAA submission to EMA via CP - its request for appointment of Rapporteur and Co-Rapporteur. This request for appointment of Rapporteur and Co-Rapporteur should be sent at least seven months prior to the intended submission date (target dates for submission of the application are published on the EMA Website[14]) of MAA to the EMA. The final appointment of the Rapporteur and Co-Rapporteur takes place six months prior to the intended submission date. The names of the Rapporteur and Co-Rapporteur will be communicated to the applicant.

The "Rapporteur" and "Co-Rapporteur" are the main responsible persons for the scientific evaluation of the MA dossier. They issue the preliminary Assessment Report (AR) which is distributed to the CHMP members and the applicant. This AR will be discussed during the next CHMP meeting and additional comments of other members of the CHMP and the outstanding issues which the applicant should address will be identified. A consolidated list of questions identifying "major objections" and/or "other concerns" may be adopted. These will be sent to the applicant together with the CHMP recommendation and scientific discussion. The clock will be stopped at this point.

---

[14] *EMA Website (http://www.emea.eu.int/ – Human Medicines - Application procedures - 'Pre-Submission Guidance')*
http://www.ema.europa.eu/ema/index.jsp?curl=pages/regulation/general/general_content_0001
19.jsp&murl=menus/regulations/regulations.jsp&mid=WC0b01ac0580022974

On or before day 210 (after answering all open issues), the CHMP adopts its opinion in the light of a final recommendation of the Rapporteur and Co-Rapporteur and further evidence presented at the oral explanation.

The draft opinion is prepared by the EMA and then adopted by the CHMP.

The CHMP opinion, which may be favorable or unfavorable, is, wherever possible, reached by scientific consensus and is the conclusion of the scientific evaluation of the CHMP. The CHMP opinion is transmitted to the European Commission (EC) within 15 days after of adoption of the opinion. Within 15 days the EC will then issue the draft Commission Decision. MSs have then 22 days to comment on the draft Commission Decision and afterwards the EC is requested to adopt a final commission Decision within 15 days. The Commission Decision leads to one single Community MA valid throughout the EU.

The Community MA confers the same rights and obligations in each of the MS as a MA granted by a MS.

For Norway and Iceland, an identical national MA will be granted subsequent to the Commission Decision.

Details of the procedure including detailed timetables can be found in the NtA VOLUME 2A - "Procedures for marketing authorisation - CHAPTER 4 - Centralised Procedure".[15]

3.2.2.3 Mutual Recognition Procedure

The legal basis for the MRP is provided in Directive 2001/83[3]. The directive is supported by some guidance documents. Detailed information on the legal basis, the scope, the requirements and the procedures are described in VOLUME 2 A NtA "Procedures for marketing authorisation CHAPTER 1 Marketing Authorisation"[12] and Volume 2 A of the NtA "Procedures for marketing authorisation - CHAPTER 2 - Mutual Recognition".[16] Some more information and guidance can be found in the "Best practice guide for decentralized and mutual recognition procedures."[17]

---

[15] *VOLUME 2A NtA - Procedures for marketing authorisation - CHAPTER 4 - Centralised Procedure from April 2006*
http://ec.europa.eu/enterprise/pharmaceuticals/eudralex/vol2/a/chap4rev200604%20.pdf

[16] *VOLUME 2A Notice to applicants - Procedures for marketing authorisation - CHAPTER 2 - Mutual Recognition from February 2007*
http://ec.europa.eu/enterprise/pharmaceuticals/eudralex/vol-2/a/vol2a_chap2_2007-02.pdf
Dated 22.07.2009

[17] *Best practice guide for decentralised and mutual recognition procedures, October 1996, revision May 2007 (CMD – Coordination group for mutual recognition procedures and decentralized procedures – human)*
http://www.hma.eu/fileadmin/dateien/Human_Medicines/CMD_h_/procedural_guidance/Application_for_MA/BPG_MRP_DCP_2007_05_Rev6_Clean.pdf

The MRP is applicable for medicinal products which already have a MA in at least one EU MS. For medicinal products with no MA in an EU MS the DCP must be used alternatively. The MRP can be used for the majority of conventional medicinal products and may also be applicable for line extensions under certain circumstances.

The MRP cannot be used for products which have been authorized via CP, but the MRP can be used for medicinal products approved under the former ex-concertation procedure and medicinal products which have been subject of a Community referral under article 30 or 31 of Directive 2001/83[3]. The MRP can also be used for generic products for which the reference product was authorized via CP.

By using the MRP the applicant intends to have an existing national MA recognized by one or more EU MSs selected by the applicant. The applicant submits identical dossiers to all relevant MSs, the so-called Concerned Member States (CMSs).

The applicant can choose one of the EU MS as Reference Member State (RMS) for the MRP. To be able to make the decision of the RMS the applicant will consider the factors like the processing time taken by each national authority, the reputation of the authority as well as the willingness of the authority to co-operate. It is advisable that the applicant discusses the proposed MAA with the RMS before submission of the dossier.

The applicants submit the MAA to the MS, which is intended to act as RMS. It is important to inform the MS that the submission will be the basis for other submissions under the MRP. Before the MRP will be initiated the applicant has to discuss the content of the Summary
of Product Characteristics (SPC), package leaflet and labeling with the RMS.

The initial MA in the RMS has to be granted within a period of 210 days after receipt of valid application. It could happen that the time period includes a clock stop in which the applicant has to submit additional requested information. The RMS evaluates the MAA dossier and prepares an AR. Before starting the MRP the applicant asks the RMS to prepare or update the AR within 90 days of receipt of this request. The AR together with the approved SPC), labeling and Patient Information Leaflet (PIL) are sent to the CMSs and the applicant by the RMS.

After receipt of the initial MA of the RMS the applicant also submits the MAA dossier to the CMSs. This dossier includes a statement that the dossier is identical to the information provided in support of the initial MAA as well as the approved SPC, labeling and PIL. Each CMS has the obligation to recognize the MA granted by the RMS within a period of 90 days. This 90 day period started after CMSs have received the AR of the RMS and have validated the application. The RMS sets the starting date of the 90 day period and informs the CMSs and the applicant respectively. [3]

If CMSs agrees to the evaluation and the AR of the RMS the procedure will be closed at day 90.

If agreement cannot be reached by the MSs, then the following stages occur:

- Reconciliation phase occurs under the direction of the Coordination group for mutual recognition procedures and decentralized procedures – human (CMD(h)) for resolution.
- If the matter cannot be resolved by the CMD then the CHMP will arbitrate and issue an option.
- CHMP opinion sent to EC.
- Commission Decision making process (EC will issue a Commission Decision based on the received CHMP opinion).

At the end of the MRP the AR is updated and national MAs are issued. The national DRAs of the CMSs have a 30 day period after finalization of the MRP to adopt the decision and issue the MA subject to the receipt of acceptable translations of the PIL. [3]

3.2.2.4 Decentralized Procedure

The legal basis for the DCP is provided in Directive 2001/83[3]. The directive is supported by some guidance documents. Detailed information on the legal basis, the scope, the requirements and the procedures are described in VOLUME 2 A NtA "Procedures for marketing authorisation CHAPTER 1 Marketing Authorisation"[12] and Volume 2 A of the NtA "Procedures for marketing authorisation - CHAPTER 2 - Mutual Recognition"[16]. The guidelines are issued with respect to the MRP but are currently also applicable for the DCP unless specific guidelines exist for the DCP or MRP guidelines cannot be used for, by similarity, for the DCP. Some more information and guidance can be also found in the "Best practice guide for decentralised and mutual recognition procedures."[17]

The DCP is open for medicinal products, which are not yet approved in any EU MS at the time of application. The DCP offers an alternative to the MRP. The DCP cannot be used for products, which have to be authorized via CP, but the DCP can be used for duplicate applications and extension applications of products originally approved by the MRP. In addition it is possible to use the DCP for generic products for which the reference product was authorized via CP.

The main difference between MRP and DCP is the fact that the initial MA is not submitted and issued for the RMS alone. Instead of this, the MAA dossier is submitted to the RMS and the CMSs (all EU MS where the MA is sought) in parallel. A statement that the identical dossier is submitted to RMS and CMSs is submitted together with the MAA dossier. The RMS will prepare a draft AR in consultation with the CMSs. This AR is the basis for the RMS and CMSs to agree the terms for the MA.

The applicant can choose one of the EU MS as RMS for the DCP. To be able to make a decision on the RMS the applicant will consider the factors like the reputation of the DRA, the willingness of the authority to co-operate as well as processing time taken by each national DRA. It is advisable that the applicant discusses the proposed MAA with the RMS at least two months before submission of the dossier.

The DCP involves the following stages and takes at maximum 210 days (for more information please refer to Volume 2A NtA "Procedures for marketing authorization - Chapter 2")[16]:

- Marketing Authorization Holder (MAH) initiates the procedure.
- Assessment Step 1:
  - RMS prepares preliminary AR, which is used for discussion between RMS, CMSs and the applicant.
  - The procedure may close if mutual consent is achieved.
- Assessment Step 2:
  - Based on draft AR, further consideration takes places between RMS and CMSs.
  - A break-out session of the MS concerned may be used for facilitation.
- If consensus cannot be reached by the MS then the following stages take place:
  - Referral to CMD for resolution.
  - If the matter cannot be resolved by the CMD then the CHMP will arbitrate and issue an option.
  - CHMP opinion sent to EC.
  - Commission Decision making process (EC will issue a Commission Decision based on the received CHMP opinion).

If agreement can be achieved after assessment step 1 the procedure takes 120 days, if assessment step 2 is needed this step will take additional 90 days, so that in total the procedure takes 210 days.

At the end of the procedure, national MAs are issued (same as done in the MRP).

3.3 USA

3.3.1 Dossier Format – ICH CTD

As described already in the section "3.1 ICH" the format for submissions in all three ICH regions, including USA is the ICH CTD format.
The ICH CTD format is applicable for Modules 2 – 5, only Module 1 differs from region to region (please refer to section "3.3.2. Dossier requirements").

3.3.2 Dossier Requirements

As mentioned in the section "3.2.1. Format and content of a Marketing Authorization Application Dossier – Regulatory Requirements" most of the dossier requirements are identical for the three ICH regions. As mentioned before the content from Module 2 – 5 is quite similar for all three ICH regions.
Nevertheless, each region has some special requirements, which are only applicable for one region.
The FDA in USA under federal law regulates the NDA and the biologics license application (BLA) process. The FDA Center for Drug Evaluation and Research (CDER) is responsible for the review of the NDAs and for parts of the BLAs.[18]

CDER is responsible for the regulatory review and supervision of drug applications and[18]:

- MAbs for in-vivo use
- Cytokines, growth factors, enzymes, immunomodulators; and thrombolytics
- Proteins intended for therapeutic use that are extracted from animals or microorganisms, including recombinant versions of these products (except clotting factors)
- Other non-vaccine therapeutic immunotherapies

The BLA review process is handled by two different divisions of FDA, the Center for Biologics Evaluation and Research (CBER) and the CDER. The CBER is responsible for the regulatory review and supervision of:[18]

- Viral-vectored gene insertions (i.e., "gene therapy")
- Products composed of human or animal cells or from physical parts of those cells
- Allergen patch tests
- Allergenics

---

[18] http://www.fda.gov/

- Antitoxins, antivenins, and venoms
- In vitro diagnostics
- Vaccines, including therapeutic vaccines
- Toxoids and toxins intended for immunization
- Blood, blood components and related products

NDAs and BLAs can be submitted either as paper submission or electronically to the CDER or CBER.

The NDA contains all data collected during the development of a new drug whereas a BLA contains all data assembled during the development of a biological product. The NDA and BLA contain also all data from preclinical and clinical studies, which were already submitted through the Investigational New Drug (IND) process. The content of an NDA and BLA may differ based on the nature or class of the drug or the biological product.[18]

Three copies of the application are requested for NDAs and Abbreviated New Drug Application(s) (ANDA(s)) which differ in their intended purpose and therefore in content:[19]

- An archival copy
- A review copy
- A field copy

For BLAs it is requested only to submit archival and review copies, so no field copy is requested.

The archival copy includes the entire submission and is the "official" complete copy of the application whereas review and field copy request only parts of the complete submission. The archival copy acts as the official archive of the application and may be used during the review of the application.[19]

The archival copy includes the following information:

- A cover letter to:
  - confirm any agreements made between the FDA and the applicant
  - identification one or more people the FDA may contact
  - any other important information about the application

---

[19] *Federal Register Vol. 68, No. 72, April 15, 2003 – Draft Guidance - Guidance for Industry- submitting MAs according to the ICH CTD format http://edocket.access.gpo.gov/2003/pdf/03- 8802.pdf 18248 - Federal Register / Vol. 68, No. 72 / Tuesday, April 15, 2003 / Notices*

- Application Form FDA 356h serves as a cover sheet for the submission. It contains the applicant, the drug product, and indicates the applicant's intention to comply with applicable laws and regulations.

- All INDs, drug master files (DMFs) and other applications referenced in the application should be identified in the form.

- The FDA recommends using the following format:
    - The submission content should be organized and labeled as described in Form FDA 356h (4/06)[20]. This form gives a comprehensive list of each section requested in the NDA, ANDA or BLA.

The review and field copies require only a portion of the application.

- Review copies are precise duplicates of the technical sections of the archival copy. They include the information needed by each review discipline for its evaluation. These copies facilitate the concurrent review of the application by the different review disciplines.

Review copies that may be necessary according to Title 21, Code of Federal Regulations (CFR) part 314.50[21] for an individual submission includes:

- Quality (Module 3),

- Nonclinical (Module 4),

- Clinical (Module 5) - safety and efficacy documents for clinical reviewer,

- Clinical (Module 5) - safety and efficacy documents for the statistical reviewer,

- Clinical (Module 5) - clinical pharmacology and pharmacokinetics documents (or bioequivalence documents for ANDAs), and

- Clinical (Module 5) – clinical microbiology documents.

---

[20] *Form FDA-356h "Application to market a new drug, biologic or an antibiotic drug for human use" (Title 21, Code of Federal Regulations parts 314 and 610)*
http://www.fda.gov/opacom/morechoices/fdaforms/internal/FDA-356h.pdf
[21] *Code of Federal Regulations, Title 21 – Foods and Drugs, Volume 5, Revised as of April 1, 2008 (CITE: 21 CFR 314.50)*
http://www.accessdata.fda.gov/scripts/cdrh/cfdocs/cfcfr/CFRSearch.cfm?fr=314.50
*Chapter 1 – Food and drugs administration department of health and human services
Subchapter D – drugs for human use
Part 314 – Applications for FDA approval to market a new drug
Subpart B – Applications; Section 314.50 – Content and format of an application*

A copy of Modules 1 and 2 should be included in each review copy including a ToC for the section, cover letter, a copy of the application form, any letter of reference or authorization, index to the entire application and the application summary. Each review copy should be labeled and bound separately.

The applicant should contact the office with the responsibility for the review of its product to determine how many copies of each module or sections of modules should be submitted.[19]

The field copy which is used by FDA inspectors during pre-approval manufacturing inspections is a copy of the Quality section (Module 3) plus form FDA 356h and the NDA summary. The field copy is only requested for the NDA and ANDA (not for BLAs). This separately bound copy should be sent directly to the appropriate field office.[19]

The "Guidance for Industry-submitting MAs according to the ICH CTD format"[19] describes the US typical documents and their content. The content of the CTD sections is not in the scope of this guidance document.
Besides the usual CTD sections, which are requested for all ICH regions the additional documents, are requested for an NDA or BLA in USA[19] which are listed in appendix 4 ("APPENDIX 4: Table of contents for an NDA in USA ").

3.3.3 Registration Procedures

As mentioned before all NDAs are submitted to CDER. The Federal Regulation requests that FDA makes a final decision for an NDA within 180 days beginning with the date of filing.

After submission to CDER the CDERs Central Document Room first handled the NDAs and sent them afterwards to the appropriate review divisions.[18]

The group of reviewers (each with a different technical specialty) checking the NDA makes several decisions within 45 days after receipt of NDA. They decide whether the NDA will be filed or refused and whether the NDA will have a standard or priority review. According to the goals of the Prescription Drug User Fee Act (PDUFA) III, 90% of BLAs and NDAs filed during 2003 and 2007 have to be reviewed within 10 months after submission for standard review procedure and within 6 months for priority review applications.

In case an NDA is subject to refuse-to-file (RTF), FDA has 60 days from receipt of the NDA to inform the applicant. The RTF letter must include the reason for the refusal. In order to get an RTF NDAs must have serious deficiencies or issues.

The applicant may send a written request to FDA for an informal conference within 30 days of receipt of the RTF in case the RTF is based on defaults, duplications or incorrect format. If the RTF is based on licensing requirements the applicant have the opportunity to amend the application and resubmit it.[18]

CDER or CBER may require a pre-approval inspection of the manufacturing facilities and clinical trial sites during the review procedure of the NDA or BLA. Normally these pre-approval inspections take place in parallel to the review of the content of NDAs and BLAs. The pre-approval inspection of the manufacturing sites and clinical trial sites, which can be announced or unannounced, have the purpose to check the compliance with GMP and the consistence with the information provided in NDA/BLA. During these inspections samples of medicinal product may be collected for analysis by CDER or CBER.

Additional to the pre-approval inspection o manufacturing sites other types of inspections might be carried out and can influence the NDA/BLA review process. These inspections are conducted by the CDER's Biosearch Monitoring Program and can include: drug sponsors, clinical investigators, institutional review boards (IRBs) and contract research organizations (CROs).[18]

Review at CDER

When the NDA is submitted, it is forwarded to one of CDER's drug review divisions, which is responsible for the therapeutic class responsible for this kind of application.

During the first review phase an evaluation of the relevant parts of the application is performed by the responsible review functions which are medical, biopharmaceutical, pharmacology, statistical, chemistry and microbiology reviewers.

Each reviewer makes an assessment of the submission in his/her area of expertise. After the review a written evaluation with conclusions and recommendations is issued by each reviewer. The written evaluation of each reviewer is forwarded to the division director or to the office director. He/She checks the conclusions and recommendations of each reviewer and decides on the actions to be taken on the submission. The outcome is that one of the action letters, i.e. approval letter, approvable letter or not approvable letter, is issued. The FDA has the possibility to use Advisory Committees throughout the review process.[18]

The following steps are identical for CBER and CDER and are described under the headline "Review at CDER or CBER".[18]

Review at CBER

For an application submitted to CBER, FDA is requested to tight review timelines and performance goals based on PDUFA. These timelines are only applicable for biological products for which user fees have to be paid, but CBER tries to review also "non-user-fee" applications within the same timelines. They have also some additional goals like meet the set timelines for responding to industry requests for meetings, providing meeting minutes of health authority meetings to industry or communication of results of review if sponsor responses to clinical hold.[18]

The following steps are identical for CBER and CDER and are described under the headline "Review at CDER or CBER".[18]

Review at CDER or CBER

Due to the US regulations the FDA is asked to inform the applicant as fast as possible of:

- Deficiencies - which are easy to correct - particularly those contained in the CMC and the control sections
- Insufficient data in any of the sections
- Technical changes requested to facilitate review.

This is done by an information request letter. In case of major scientific issues, this has to be addressed in a formal action letter.

This procedure was established in order to allow the applicants to submit supplements as early as possible during the review process and before the review period is finalized. The next step in the review process is the so-called "Ninety-Day Conference". FDA will invite applicants to a review meeting approximately 90 days after receipt of the submission in order to discuss the status of review, to mention the deficiencies and to discuss other issues of mutual interest. In case a personal meeting cannot be arranged this meeting can be replaced by a telephone conference if both parties agree.

As prerequisite for approval of an application, the FDA will check whether the medicinal product meets the relevant legal standards. Depending on the type of application the legal standards are:[18]

- In the case of full applications, these standards include requirements for safety, efficacy, manufacturing controls, and labeling.
- In the case of abbreviated applications, these standards include requirements for manufacturing controls, labeling, and bioequivalence (if applicable).

It is advisable that applicants look at FDA guidelines, recommendations and policy statements to assist in submitting NDAs and BLAs.

The FDA notifies the applicant via an action letter if the product has been approved (approval letter) or unapproved (complete response letter) at the end of the review period.

There are in principle three types of letters, which FDA can issue: approval letter, approvable letter, and not approvable letter.

The FDA will issue a not approvable letter if they believe that the NDA cannot be approved. Within the not approvable letter any deficiencies in the NDA are described. The applicant will respond to a not approvable letter within 10 days of the date of the letter for full applications in one of the following forms:[18]

- Resubmit (i.e. a formal response to the action letter) or acknowledge the intent to file a resubmission to the NDA or BLA

- Request for a reasonable extension of the review period to be able to provide the appropriate response

- Request for a hearing

Before the FDA finalizes the review cycle and issues an approval letter they may request more data or ask for a clarification about existing data or some other element in the NDA/BLA. In such a case FDA will issue an approvable letter. With issuing an approvable letter FDA believes that the NDA or BLA can be approved once the applicant will provide the additional requested information or agrees on specific conditions (like changes in labeling). The approvable letter will describe the additional information requested by FDA or the conditions to which the applicant have to agree in order to obtain the approval.

The approvable letter will be answered by the applicant within 10 days of the date of the letter or number of days specified in the letter in one of the following forms:[18]

- Resubmit (i.e. a formal response to the action letter) or acknowledge the intent to make a resubmission to the NDA or BLA

- Request for a hearing

- Withdrawal of the application

- Request for a reasonable extension of the review period in order to be able to provide the appropriate response to the approvable letter. When an extension is granted, the applicant must respond within the agreed time period. If not done, FDA will consider the application as withdrawn.

As mentioned above FDA has also the possibility to issue a complete response letter. Such a letter is issued if FDA will not approve the NDA, ANDA or BLA in its present form for one or more reasons. This procedure is laid down in revised 21 CFR Part

314.110 effective August 11, 2008[22]. Within the complete response letter all deficits, which FDA has identified during the review cycle within the application for not approving the product, are mentioned. If possible FDA will also recommend further actions for the application in order to put the application in place for conditions for approval.[18]

In case FDA asks for Phase IV studies all agreements regarding the schedule and nature of the Phase IV study will be mentioned in the approval letter.

If FDA approves a medicinal product the product can be put on the market. As soon as the product is approved for marketing FDA is obliged to make some research information from applicant available to public, which were evaluated through the experts of CDER or CBER. These documents are referred to as Drug Approval packages (formerly known as Summary Basis for approval). The drug approval package contains the rational for approving the medicinal product. In addition, it contains the approval letter, professional labeling, PIL and the reviews from the CBER or CDER reviewers (e.g., medical, chemistry, pharmacology, clinical, statistical, etc) as well as administrative Information and correspondence. This information can be made available through the Freedom of Information (FOI) Act per 21 CFR Part 20[23]. These drug approval packages contain normally between 50 – 1500 pages. To make the handling of these approval packages more comfortable FDA prepares a ToC and identifies the pivotal studies of the medicinal product. The pivotal studies are the essential studies for the application on which basis the efficacy and safety of the medicinal product can be proven. Abstracts of the pivotal studies are also included in the ToC.[18]

Other registration procedures

FDA has established three formal procedures to accelerate the development and review process. These procedures are applicable for drugs and biologics that address unmet medical need or for serious life-threatening diseases or conditions.[24]

These three procedures are fast track product development, priority review and accelerated approval.

Accelerated Approval

---

[22] *Code of Federal Regulations, Title 21 – 21 CFR Part 314.110 effective August 11, 2008* http://edocket.access.gpo.gov/2008/pdf/E8-15610.pdf and http://law.justia.com/us/cfr/title21/21-5.0.1.1.4.4.1.10.html dated 01.09.2009

[23] *Freedom of Information (FOI) Act per 21 CFR Part 20 (cf. XXX)* http://www.fda.gov/AboutFDA/ReportsManualsForms/StaffManualGuides/ucm138408.htm - dated 01.09.2009

[24] Susan Thaul, *FDA Fast Track and Priority Review Programs, CRS Report of Congress - Order Code RS22814*, February 21, 2008 http://www.nationalaglawcenter.org/assets/crs/RS22814.pdf - dated 01.09.2009

FDA regulations, published in 1992, allow "accelerated approval" for drugs or biologics products which provide meaningful therapeutic benefit...over existing treatments. This type of procedure is applicable for the treatment of a serious or life-threatening disease.

The procedure allows the approval based on clinical trials using "a surrogate endpoint that is reasonable likely... to predict clinical benefit." instead of using standard outcome measures like survival or disease progression.

Another possibility for the use of this procedure are drugs for which the use could be considered safe and effective only under set restrictions which could include limited prescribing or dispensing. For these types of drugs FDA normally requires postmarketing studies after the approval.[24]

Fast-Track Mechanism

The Food and Drug Administration Modernization Act of 1997 (FDAMA, P.L. 105-115)[25] directed the secretary to create a mechanism whereby FDA could designate as "Fast Track".

The "Fast track" is designed for certain products that met two criteria:

- The product must concern a serious or life-threatening condition

- It has to have the potential to address an unmet medical need

The two main goals of the fast track are on the one hand making approval more likely and on the other hand the shortening of the approval time.

After FDA has granted a fast track designation the manufacturer is encouraged to meet with the FDA in order to discuss development plans and strategies before the official submission of the NDA/BLA. The advantage of the early interaction with FDA is that issues like elements of clinical study designs and presentations whose absence at NDA/BLA can lead to a delay in approval decision of NDA/BLA can be clarified earlier.[24]

On the other hand, FDA offers similar interactions to any sponsor who asks for FDA consultation throughout the development phases of a medicinal product. A unique option within Fast Track is the opportunity of a rolling submission, i.e. to submit sections of an NDA/BLA to FDA as they are ready, rather than the standard requirement to submit a complete application at one time.[24]

---

[25]*Food and Drug Administration Modernization Act of 1997 (FDAMA, P.L. 105-115)*
http://www.fda.gov/RegulatoryInformation/Legislation/FederalFoodDrugandCosmeticActFDCAct
/SignificantAmendmentstotheFDCAct/FDAMA/FullTextofFDAMAlaw/default.htm - dated 22.10.2009

Priority Review

In comparison to the fast track or accelerated approval, the priority review process starts only when a manufacturer officially submits an NDA/BLA.

Therefore the priority review does not have any influence on the timing or content of steps taken during the drug development or the testing of safety and efficacy.

The priority review can be used for medicinal products, which are intended to address unmet medical need. In such a case the duration of review (NDA/BLA) can be shortened from 10 months (full review time for a normal NDA/BLA) to 6 months (priority review of NDA/BLA). The priority review is not explicitly required by law, but FDA has established it in practice, and various statutes, such as the PDUFA, refer to and sometimes require it.

In appendix 5 an overview table with the comparison of mechanisms to hasten product availability is attached ("APPENDIX 5: Table of Comparison of Mechanisms to Hasten Product Availability").[24]

The accelerated approval, fast track mechanism and priority review are not described here in more details.

3.4 CADREAC
3.4.1 General Information

The **C**ollaboration **A**greement of **D**rug **R**egulatory Authorities in **E**uropean **U**nion **A**ssociated **C**ountries (CADREAC) was a collaboration of countries, which started in 1997. The Heads of DRAs in the EU associated countries agreed to sign the CADREAC agreement in order to start a formal collaboration during the first meeting of DRAs in Central and Eastern Europe Countries (CEECs), 12 to 14 June 1997 in Sofia.[26]

Up to April 2007, 13 state regulatory authorities for human medicinal products of countries in Central, Eastern and Southern Europe had signed the CADREAC agreement:

- Bulgaria, Czech Republic, Estonia, Hungary, Latvia, Lithuania, Poland, Romania, Slovakia (since 1997)
- Slovenia (since 1998)
- Cyprus (since 1999)
- Turkey (since 2001)
- Croatia (since 2005)

---

[26] http://www.dgra.de/studiengang/pdf/master_hoerner_a.pdf - dated 22.10.2009

Nine of the original CADREAC countries (Cyprus, Czech Republic, Estonia, Hungary, Latvia, Lithuania, Poland, Slovakia and Slovenia) joined the EU at 1st May 2004 and two other countries (Bulgaria and Romania) joined the EU at 1st January 2007, therefore in April 2007 there were only two CADREAC states left – Croatia and Turkey. The mission of CADREAC was facilitation of smooth transition of regulatory conditions in EU associated countries to achieve regulatory standards required by Acquis Communautaire (compliance to article (Art.) 6 of Directive 2001/83/EEC[3] amended by Directive 2004/27[4]: *"No medicinal product may be placed on the market of a Member State unless a marketing authorisation has been issued by the competent authorities of that Member State in accordance with this Directive or an authorisation has been granted in accordance with Regulation (EEC) No 2309/93. The authorisation referred to in paragraph 1 shall also be required for radionuclide generators, radionuclide kits, radionuclide precursor radiopharmaceuticals and industrially prepared radiopharmaceuticals."*, which are:

- Implementation of EU regulatory standards
- Involvement in professional activities within EU
- Introduction of MRP
- Introduction of CP
- Development of common strategies
- Preparation of meetings
- Information exchange

A CADREAC Standard Operating Procedure (SOP), CADREAC SOP-3 (2001) was adopted in April 2001, defining the responsibilities and function of a CADREAC secretariat.[27]

The DRA, which acted as CADREAC secretariat, was selected at CADREAC annual assembly at least one year before the term of service.

The activities of the CADREAC secretariat started with the organization of CADREAC annual meeting, including drafting of the agenda and minutes of CADREAC annual meeting. The activities ended with drafting and presenting CADREAC annual report to be approved at CADREAC annual meeting and with providing all necessary information to its successor.

If no other delegation was made, CADREAC secretariat was the principle contact point for CADREAC.

---

[27] *CADREAC SOP: CADREAC SOP-3 (2001) - Responsibilities and function of CADREAC secretariat http://old.sukl.cz/en06/en0601.htm*

The CADREAC secretariat was also responsible for:

- Maintenance of CADREAC documents, especially keeping lists updated of
  - CADREAC agreed documents (like Common procedures, SOPs, positions) except Collaboration Agreement
  - DRAs – CADREAC members and observers to CADREAC
  - CADREAC observers at European Community/EMA working parties and committees
  - CADREAC experts serving as contact points for sending materials from working parties
- Co-ordination of distribution of relevant information, esp. drafts and final versions of CADREAC documents and co-ordination of activities needed to obtain common CADREAC opinion
- Prepare documents to be published on the CADREAC homepage

The secretariat of CADREAC is located in Romania since March 2004.
In addition to the CADREAC MSs, the following countries had the status of observers: Belarus, Bosnia-Herzegovina, Republic of Moldova, CH and Serbia and Montenegro.
The CADREAC countries developed certain guidelines and procedures as a preparation for their EU-accession.
A number of procedures and agreed documents have been published in the internet[28]:

- Common procedure on the granting of MAs by CADREAC DRAs for medicinal products authorized in the EU by CP - in force since January 1999[6]
- Common procedure on the granting of MAs by CADREAC DRAs for medicinal products authorized in the EU by MRP - in force since May 2001 (The 1st revision of the guideline - published June 10th, 2001 - includes the retrospective inclusion of medicinal products for human use authorized in EU via MRP in the Common CADREAC Simplified System)[7]
- Common CADREAC Procedure (CCP) for retrospective inclusion of centrally authorized medicinal products for human use in the Common CADREAC Simplified System - in force since May 2001 [29]
- SOPs
- Lists of contact points

---

[28] *CADREAC homepage - http://web.archive.org/web/20040605093650/http://www.cadreac.org*
[29] *Common CADREAC Procedure (CCP) for retrospective inclusion of centrally authorized medicinal products for human use in the Common CADREAC Simplified System - in force since May 2001 http://www.milray.org/pdf/CADREAC.pdf*

- Lists of CADREAC observers in European Community/EMA working parties and of observers to CADREAC

During the initial CADREAC initiative it was possible since January 1st, 2002 to use the CADREAC procedure for products authorized in EU via CP in Turkey even if Turkey was not a full member of CADREAC. The use of this simplified CADREAC procedure for products authorized via CP was restricted only to biotechnological products except for immunological and blood products in Turkey. Turkey did not join the CADREAC procedure for products authorized in EU via MRP.

As most of the "old" CADREAC countries have meanwhile joined the EU on May 1st, 2004, the CADREAC initiative was dissolved. Therefore a subsequent initiative was established. This new initiative is called new CADREAC or nCADREAC (New Collaboration Agreement between Drug Regulatory Authorities in Central and Eastern European Countries). This new initiative has also established a CADREAC agreement, which was signed on 1st May 2005.

The active members of this new CADREAC initiative are Bulgaria, Croatia, Czech Republic, Hungary, Romania and Slovak Republic. Collaborative members are Kosovo and Republic of Moldova.[30] Further information can be found on the homepage of nCADREAC initiative: http://www.newcadreac.org/[30].

The CADREAC secretariat is still at the Romanian health authority "National Medicines Agency" and has nearly the same responsibilities as in the original CADREAC initiative. The nCADREAC procedures which are nearly identical to the originally CADREAC procedures were released on January 10th, 2006.[31, 32]

The nCADREAC procedures were only applicable for Bulgaria, Romania and Croatia as all other active members were already EU member states and Turkey which in the past only attended the CADREAC procedure for CP authorized products is no part of nCADREAC anymore. After the EU accession of Bulgaria and Romania on January 1st, 2007 the nCADREAC procedure remains for Croatia and other potential accession countries. The nCADREAC procedure for CP authorized products[31] can only be used in Bulgaria, Croatia and Romania and not in Turkey anymore. The nCADREAC procedure

---

[30] http://www.newcadreac.org/members.html

[31] *Procedure on the granting of marketing authorisations by new CADREAC (nCADREAC) drug regulatory authorities for medicinal products for human use already authorised in EU member states following the centralized procedure and the variation and renewal of such marketing authorisations*

[32] *Procedure on the granting of marketing authorisations by new CADREAC (nCADREAC) drug regulatory authorities for medicinal products for human use already authorised in EU member states following the mutual recognition procedure and the variation and renewal of such marketing authorisations*

for products authorized via MRP is also only possible in Bulgaria, Croatia and Romania.[32]

3.4.2 Dossier Format – ICH CTD

In the CADREAC countries also the ICH CTD is used as format (please refer to section 3.1 ICH).

3.4.3 Dossier Requirements

The dossier requirements for nCADREAC countries are based on EU requirements as their regulations and procedures are based on EU regulations. Therefore the principle regulatory requirements for getting an MAA within the EU - which are described in the NtA Volume 2B: "Medicinal products for human use - Presentation and format of the dossier Common Technical Document (CTD)"[10] - are also valid for nCADREAC countries, like Croatia.

Additionally to the CTD dossier (Module 2 - 5) some Module 1 documents are required. For Croatia, as one example of an nCADREAC country, the following Module 1 requirements are requested (depending whether the reference product is authorized via CP or MRP/DCP):

- For MRP/DCP[7, 32] authorized products if submission is done in nCADREAC country after finalization of MRP/CDP:

  - *"Application form (the appropriate national application form for the marketing authorisation of a medicinal product together with administrative data and samples required by the nCADREAC DRA concerned)*

  - *Dossier identical with the dossier submitted in the EU-CMSs in MRP*

  - *Consolidated list of questions raised by CMSs within the MRP and Applicant response document in MRP (day 65 responses to questions raised by CMSs within the MRP) and later responses*

  - *Updated Assessment Report (UAR) of RMS, including harmonised SPC (if European DMF Procedure has been used, the assessment report on the restricted part should be requested from RMS directly)*

  If there is only RMS Assessment Report available, the applicant should provide information on the MRP:

  - *list of CMSs*

  - *history of the MRP*

- *break out session minutes, if applicable*
- *information about the reasons for withdrawal(s)*
- *the letter of RMS about the completion of the procedure (first use, repeat use) with SPC attached*
- *In case that variations have been accepted after conclusion of the MRP, a list of these variations has to be part of the submission; the documentation submitted in the EU-MSs to support these variations shall be annexed to the original dossier*
- *variation assessment report(s), if applicable*
- *the letter of RMS about the completion of the variation procedure with SPC attached*
- *In case the application in the nCADREAC concerned candidate countries (nC-CCC) is submitted later than 9 months after the authorisation in EU-RMS and concerns a new active substance, the latest available PSUR (Period Safety Update Report)*
- *List of post-authorisation commitments imposed in MRP and the status of their fulfillment, if any*
- *Declaration of the applicant that*
  - *he will deal with nCADREAC DRA concerned similarly as he or relevant MAH deals with DRAs of EU-MSs, especially he will keep the product authorised by the nCADREAC DRA concerned identical with the EU-MSs, i.e. in the post-authorisation phase he will notify and implement all urgent safety measures simultaneously in the EU-MSs and the nC-CCCs and he will submit and implement all variations, once accepted in the EU-MSs, without unnecessary delay*
  - *dossier submitted to the nC-CCC is identical to the dossier submitted in the EU-CMSs for MRP, including all information submitted to support any variation which has been applied for and accepted at the time of submission of the application in the nC-CCC as well as information concerning post-authorisation commitments, if any (i.e. the documentation reflects the situation of the product, which is in the EU-MSs at the time of submission of the application in the nC-CCC)*
  - *the submitted proposal of SPC in local language is the translation of SPC as last approved in MRP*

- *Declaration of the MAH in RMS and if necessary, also of the holder of restricted part of DMF (see Annex 1). "*

The evaluation of the dossier and the assessment procedure remain country specific. Each nCADREAC DRA will review the dossier submitted for simplified procedure individually. Based on the individual evaluation of each nCADREAC DRA, each nCADREAC DRA will create an AR and will send the report of the outcome to the RMS and a copy to the CADREAC secretariat.

- MRP/DCP[7, 32] – if submission is done in nCADREAC country during MRP/DCP:

  - *"Application form (the appropriate national application form for the marketing authorisation of a medicinal product together with administrative data and samples required by the nCADREAC DRA concerned)*

  - *Dossier identical with the dossier submitted in the EU-CMSs in MRP*

  - *Assessment Report of RMS including SPC as approved in the RMS in English language (if European DMF Procedure has been used, the assessment report on the restricted part should be requested from RMS directly)*

  - *Declaration of the applicant that:*

    - *he will deal with nCADREAC DRA concerned similarly as he or relevant MAH deals with DRAs of EU-MSs, especially he will keep the product authorised by the nCADREAC DRA concerned identical with the EU-MSs, i.e. in the post-authorisation phase he will notify and implement all urgent safety measures simultaneously in the EU-MSs and the nC-CMSs and he will submit and implement all variations, once accepted in the EU-MSs, without unnecessary delay*

    - *dossier submitted to the nCADREAC DRA concerned is identical to the dossier submitted in the RMS and EU-CMSs for MRP, if applicable*

    - *he will inform the nCADREAC DRA concerned on each step of the relevant MRP*

  - *Declaration of the MAH in RMS and if necessary, also of the holder of restricted part of DMF"*

The applicant provides the nCADREAC DRA with the information on all steps of the MRP in due time as defined for MRPs in the " Best practice guide for DCP and MRP, October 1996" as currently revised in May 2007[17].

The assessment procedure remains country specific. Each nCADREAC DRA will review the dossier submitted for simplified procedure individually.

Each nCADREAC DRA will create an AR and will send the report on the outcome to the RMS and a copy to the nCADREAC secretariat.

- $CP^{6,31}$ authorized products:

    - *"application form (the appropriate national application form for the marketing authorisation of a medicinal product)*

    - *modules 1, 2 and 3 of the dossier as accepted by the EMEA and detailed list of contents of modules 4 and 5, providing that these parts are submitted on request*

    - *proposed SPC, PIL in national language and the labelling in national language unless otherwise specified in the attached table; SPC and PIL are translations of the texts approved or in the case of earlier submission of the texts submitted in the EU without changes*

    - *final CHMP Assessment Report including all annexes (see Note below)*

    - *final Commission Decision including all annexes (see Note below)*

    - *declaration by the applicant that*

        - *the dossier submitted, or, where appropriate, the parts submitted thereof are identical to the dossier of a product authorised in the EU by the centralised procedure (in the case of an earlier submission, to be identical to the dossier submitted to EMEA), including all information submitted to support any variation which has been applied for and accepted at the time of submission of the application for marketing authorisation at the nCADREAC DRA concerned as well as information concerning post-authorisation commitments, if any*

        - *all subsequent variations to this dossier, once accepted in the EU, will also be submitted and implemented without delay by the applicant in the nC-CCC*

        - *all urgent safety measures will be immediately notified to the nCADREAC DRA concerned and implemented according to local regulatory requirements simultaneously as in the EU or as soon as possible*

- in the case where the marketing authorisation will be suspended or withdrawn in the EU (either by the initiative of the MAH or by EC), nCADREAC DRAs concerned will be notified immediately
- copy of the declaration by MAH in the EU (the Declaration is sent to the EMEA) that
  - an application is being submitted to one or more nCADREAC DRAs, indicating the countries concerned, pertaining to the name of the product, the Community Marketing Authorisation number, the MAH in the EU as well as the proposed MAH in the nC-CCC
  - he agrees that the EMEA may make available to the nCADREAC DRA concerned any information to the quality, safety and efficacy of the product concerned (the extent of this information shall not exceed that which is made available to EU MSs by the EMEA)
- list of all resolved/outstanding post-authorisation commitments
- If the application is submitted later than 6 months after the date of the Commission Decision, then the latest available Periodic Safety Update Report (PSUR), which should include any new pharmacovigilance data, shall be submitted.
  - Similarly, if any variations to the marketing authorisation in the EU have been applied for and accepted at the time of submission of the application for marketing authorisation in the nCADREAC countries, relevant details should be provided. The information submitted to the EMEA to support these variations should also be submitted in the nCADREAC DRAs concerned and may be annexed to the original dossier (see table of dossier requirements). The following documents should also be provided:
  - list of all variations to the marketing authorisation that have been approved in the EU, safety, transfer or renewal approved procedures at the time of the date of submission of the application in the nCADREAC DRAs concerned
  - Commission Decisions granting marketing authorization for the medicinal product for human use, Commission Decision amending the marketing authorisation as a consequence of an approved type II variation, Annex II application, Renewal, Annual Reassessment, transfer of the marketing authorisation or safety procedure, if issued by European Commission, as well as for an approved type IA, IB variation (every six months)

- *Notifications on a type IB variation to the terms of the marketing authorisation, issued by the EMEA;*
- *Notifications of the minor changes in labelling or package leaflet not connected with the SPC (Art. 61.3 Notification)*
- *Acknowledgement of receipt of a valid notification for type IA variation to the terms of the marketing authorization*
- *Variation assessment reports, if issued*
- *samples as specified in attached table."*

3.4.4 Registration Procedures - Example Croatia

The nCADREAC procedures relating to regulatory activities for products authorized in EU via CP is operational since January 2006 and is described in the document "Procedure on the granting of marketing authorisations by new CADREAC (nCADREAC) drug regulatory authorities for medicinal products for human use already authorised in EU member states following the centralised procedure and the variation and renewal of such marketing authorisations".[31]

The document describes the simplified CADREAC procedure for the granting of MAs by CADREAC DRAs for centrally authorized medicinal products for human use and the post-authorization activities – VARs, RENs and handling of pharmacovigilance information - of such MAs.

This simplified nCADREAC procedure for products authorized in EU via CP described in this document is optional and can only be initiated at the EU MAH`s request. This means that there is no legal obligation to use the simplified nCADREAC procedure.

The original simplified CADREAC procedure has entered into force on 1st January 1999, the nCADREAC procedure for CP authorized products has come into force dated January10th, 2006.

The procedure itself consists of the following five steps[31]:

1. "Initiation of the procedure

The EU MAH initiates the procedure and notifies the EMEA (see Annex 1) that an application will be submitted in one or more nCADREAC DRAs and indicates:

- *the nCADREAC DRA concerned*
- *the name of the product in the EU, pharmaceutical form(s), strength(s) authorised in the EU*
- *International Nonproprietary Name (INN) or common name of the active substance(s)*

- *the Community Marketing Authorisation number(s)*
- *the EU MAH*
- *the proposed MAH in the nC-CCC*
- *the proposed name of the product in the nC-CCC*

Furthermore, the EU MAH declares that the EMEA and the European Commission may make available to the nCADREAC DRA concerned any information in relation to the quality, safety and efficacy of the above medicinal product, using the form attached as Annex 1.

The EMEA subsequently includes this information in the relevant database.

2. Submission of the application

The applicant (i.e. proposed nCADREAC MAH) submits the application to the nCADREAC DRA concerned. The addresses of the nCADREAC DRAs are provided in Annex 3. Furthermore, the proposed nCADREAC MAH certifies that the application is identical with the application accepted in the EU with the exception of the following parameters, where relevant: MAH, pack sizes (not all pack sizes are necessarily authorised in nC-CCC), the name of the medicinal product (in substantiated cases only)."

3. Timing

It is possible to submit the applications either after the finalization of the EU CP (after issuing the final Commission Decision) or during the ongoing CP. This is dependent on the nCADREAC countries concerned. In case of an early submission in the nCADREAC country the applicant has to inform the nCADREAC DRAs about the submission and the successful validation of the MAA in the CP. This is done by submitting a letter from EMA informing the applicant of the positive outcome of the validation and about the adopted timetable for the CP or the CHMP opinion. The simplified nCADREAC procedure can be finalized first after the submission of the final Commission Decision to the nCADREAC DRAs. In Croatia the timing for the evaluation of the application takes according to the guideline 5 months and submission of the application is first possible after finalization of the CP.

4. "Outcome of the procedure

The nCADREAC DRA concerned informs the EMEA (the Head of Unit EMEA Post-Authorisation Evaluation of Medicines for Human Use), with copy to the applicant, at the end of the procedure on its outcome using the form provided in Annex 2.

In case of a favourable outcome (i.e. recognition of the Commission Decision granting the EU marketing authorisation), the following information will be provided:

- *name of the medicinal product in the nC-CCC*
- *national Marketing Authorisation Number(s)*
- *name of the MAH in the nC-CCC*
- *date of issue of national Marketing Authorisation*
- *authorised pharmaceutical form(s), strength(s), pack size(s)*
- *any differences between SPC, PL, and labelling approved in the nC-CCC and the EU where relevant*

In case of disagreement with the Commission Decision granting the EU marketing authorisation, the scientific conclusions which led to such disagreement are communicated.

The nCADREAC DRA concerned will also inform the other nCADREAC DRAs concerned in case of any disagreement with or modification of the Commission Decision.

5. Follow-up to the procedure

Upon receipt of information regarding the outcome of the procedure, the EMEA will include such information in the relevant database.

The EMEA will keep its scientific committee, the CHMP informed about the finalisation of any procedure which resulted in a disagreement with or modification of the Commission Decision initiated in accordance with the above described framework. Where necessary, the EMEA will inform the nCADREAC DRAs concerned of the CHMP's consideration of the issue (especially in case of disagreement with the Commission Decision)."

The guidance which describes the nCADREAC procedure for products authorized in EU via MRP (simplified nCADREAC MRP) is called "Procedure on the granting of marketing authorisations by new CADREAC (nCADREAC) drug regulatory authorities for medicinal products for human use already authorised in EU member states following the mutual recognition procedure and the variation and renewal of such marketing authorisations".[32]

The aim of this guidance which describes the nCADREAC procedure for products authorized in EU via MRP (simplified nCADREAC MRP) is the description of a procedure which can be used by each nCADREAC DRA for granting a MA of a medicinal product which has been authorized in the EU MSs following the MRP including subsequent VARs and RENs.

The simplified nCADREAC procedure offers the possibility of harmonization of SPC, PIL and documentation of medicinal products authorized in the EU MSs following the MRP with the nCADREAC MSs.

It should be also considered that harmonization of innovative products authorized by nCADREAC DRAs with those authorized in the EU is one of the conditions for harmonization of their generics in the future.[32]

The original simplified CADREAC procedure for products authorized in EU via MRP has entered into force on 3rd May 2001, whereas the simplified nCADREAC procedure for products authorized in EU via MRP is in place since January10[th], 2006.

The mentioned document[32] describing the simplified nCADREAC procedure for products authorized in EU via MRP is divided into the following sections:

- *"Principles*
- *Responsibilities of concerned parties*
- *MA procedure*
- *VARs to the MA*
- *Handling of Pharmacovigilance information*
- *RENs of MAs*
- *Annexes 1 – 4"*

Principles of the simplified nCADREAC procedure

Before starting with the description of the procedure itself the principles of the procedure and the responsibilities of the concerned parties are described for a better understanding of the procedure.

The basic principle of the nCADREAC procedure is the mutual recognition of the EU MRP, i.e. the recognition of the assessment of the RMS (and CMSs) in EU. The scope of the nCADREAC procedure is to offer a possibility of a procedure, which can be used by any nCADREAC DRA for granting a MA of a medicinal product, which has been authorized in the EU MSs following the MRP including subsequent VARs and RENs. The assessment of the RMS can be assumed to be relevant for nCADREAC area because it can be expected that differences in medical practice between the EU MSs and nCADREAC area are generally not of major importance for public health.[7,32]

The use of the nCADREAC procedure is not mandatory, but voluntary. The applicant and the nCADREAC DRAs can decide whether to use the nCADREAC procedure or not. The simplified procedure as such is initiated by the applicant (RMS MAH or headquarter of company) with the submission of an application for MA to a nCADREAC DRA with an additional procedure specific documentation.[7,32]

The nCADREAC DRA specifies individually which products could be subjects to the procedure and there are in principle three options depending on the respective country which products can be included in the nCADREAC procedure:[7,32]

1. „only products submitted for MRP in MSs with full dossier and submitted for the simplified procedure to nCADREAC DRA from CC also with full dossier and subsequently for their line extensions,
2. in addition to products mentioned under 1. also line extensions of products based on full dossier, which passed MRP, but the first product in the line is not harmonised in the country of the nCADREAC DRA concerned - simplified procedure applied on the line extension, can therefore start only after harmonisation of the first product in the line, achieved by variations,
3. all products submitted for MRP, including generics."

The applicant has to ensure the identity of the dossier and SPC submitted, as well as identical post-approval development, urgent safety measures and VARs of the product in the EU-MSs and in the countries of the nC-CCC.

The only acceptable differences in nCADREAC procedure are the name of the medicinal product and name of the MAH compared to MRP. In addition, it is not necessary to apply for all package sizes in the nC-CCC which have been applied for and which are authorized in the CMSs. Legal status of the product is based on the national regulations and the decision is made by the nC-CCC. [7,32]

The RMS has the duty to provide the updated AR to the applicant or to respective nCADREAC DRA directly.

In addition, nCADREAC DRA concerned should be provided with all necessary information also in the post-approval phase (e.g. rapid alerts, urgent safety restrictions (USRs), VARs) via the applicant or directly by the RMS, based on the declaration on information sharing of the RMS MAH. In each EU-MS and in the nCADREAC DRAs, contact points have been established for communication. [7,32]

If questions or concerns to the EU-RMS AR are raised by the nCADREAC DRA, documents in addition to the submitted dossier may be required by the nCADREAC DRA from the applicant, or additional assessment according to the usual national procedure may be carried out.

It remains a national nC-CCC decision to establish a special track for processing these MAAs in the nCADREAC DRA with possible acceleration.

National legislation of each nCADREAC country is applicable for all requirements of dossier submission, e.g. number of copies, samples, acceptance of electronic dossiers and regulation of fees. [7,32]

The nCADREAC DRAs keep their responsibilities for granting MAAs, approving VARs and RENs and supervising safety measures within their respective territories according to their national regulations and national legislations. [7,32]

Each nCADREAC DRA can decide about the starting point of the procedure. The procedure will be started after submission of the MAA to the nCADREAC DRA. There is the possibility to start the procedure at any time after completion of the respective (first) recognition procedure by the EU CMSs, i.e. after the day 90, (further on described as variant I) or to start the procedure already when the MA is granted only by the RMS (further described as variant II).

It is allowed that experts of nCADREAC DRA concerned or nCADREAC observers participate in a break-out session of MRP, based on a written agreement of the applicant in the RMS, in case that an application is pending at a nCADREAC DRA and EU-CMSs in parallel. [7,32]

The nCADREAC DRA decides whether just one or both of the described variants are practiced. The submission must comply with the administrative requirements of the nC-CCC.

All requirements for dossier submission e.g. number of copies, samples, acceptance of electronic dossiers and the regulation of fees are in the national responsibility of the nC-CCC and local legislations are applicable for these issues. The specific national requirements of each nCADREAC DRA are listed in the Annex 4 of the document - „Table of specific national requirements of nCADREAC DRAs concerned" of the document "Procedure on the granting of marketing authorisations by new CADREAC (nCADREAC) drug regulatory authorities for medicinal products for human use already authorised in EU member states following the mutual recognition procedure and the variation and renewal of such marketing authorisations"[7,32] (see APPENDIX 6).

In addition also issues like intellectual property (IP) rights and confidentiality remain in the responsibility of the nC-CCC.

It should be emphasized that variant II was in the past (at the original CADREAC procedure) only possible in Slovakia but pre-submission consultation was required. In all other nCADREAC and CADREAC (new EU-MSs) countries only variant I was and is possible – submission of the MAA any time after completion of the respective MRP, when an updated AR is available - whereas in Czech Republic, Hungary and Latvia variant I was possible after day 90 of the MRP. Therefore for most of the CADREAC and nCADREAC countries only variant I was and is feasible, i.e. for all current nCADREAC countries only variant I is accepted.

Responsibilities of the concerned parties

One other important aspect for the nCADREAC procedure are the concerned parties which are involved in the nCADREAC procedure - which are the applicant/MAH in the nCADREAC area, the MAH in the RMS, the CA of the RMS and the nCADREAC DRA - and their different jobs and responsibilities in the nCADREAC procedure.

The applicant/MAH in the nCADREAC area has to ensure that the dossier submitted is identical to the dossier submitted in the CMSs.

He has to take care that the declaration according to Annex $1^{7,32}$ (see APPENDIX 7) will be available also from restricted part of EDMF holder (manufacturer of active substance), if EDMF procedure has been used.

The applicant/MAH is responsible that the medicinal product will be kept identical in the post-marketing phase and that all information on the course of the MRP as required for variant II will be submitted to the nCADREAC DRA in time.

The MAH in the RMS has to sign a declaration on the information sharing and participation of experts of nCADREAC DRA concerned or observers in break-out sessions of the Mutual Recognition Facilitation Group (MRFG), if appropriate^{7,32} (see APPENDIX 7) and has to sent this declaration to the national authority of the RMS and a copy to the nCADREAC DRA.

The competent authority (CA) of the RMS has to make available the updated AR and if necessary post-approval information (like rapid alerts, USRs) to MAH in the EU or nCADREAC DRA directly.

RMS should provide nCADREAC DRA concerned with all necessary information also in the post-approval phase (like rapid alerts, USRs) via the applicant or directly, based on the declaration on information sharing of the RMS MAH. Contact points in each EU-MS and in the nCADREAC DRAs have been established for communication. ^{7,32}

The nCADREAC DRA concerned has to ensure to keep information submitted and generated during this procedure confidential and has the duty to send the report on the outcome of the procedure in the nC-CCC to the RMS (see APPENDIX 8) and a copy of the report to the nCADREAC secretariat. In case of disagreement or modification other than defined, the report will include a justification and will be also sent to all nCADREAC DRAs.

Description of the procedure for getting a MA

According to the document „Procedure on the granting of marketing authorisations by new CADREAC (nCADREAC) drug regulatory authorities for medicinal products for human use already authorised in EU member states following the mutual recognition procedure and the variation and renewal of such marketing authorisations"^{32} the initiation of the nCADREAC procedure is done by the RMS MAH. Practically, it is also possible that the headquarter of a company initiates the procedure, especially in cases where local affiliates are MAH in RMS. The initiator of the procedure notifies the EU-RMS that an MAA will be submitted in one or more nC-CCCs. In addition, the initiator of the procedure, RMS MAH, submits a written declaration to the DRA of the RMS wherein he declares that the DRA of the RMS may make available to the nCADREAC DRA any information regarding quality, safety and efficacy of the concerned product(s) and in the case that variant II is used he agrees with the participation of the nCADREAC expert in the break out session (see APPENDIX 7).

It should be considered, that the nCADREAC procedure itself and the evaluation of dossier are not described in detail in the nCADREAC procedure document.[7,32]

As mentioned before, the nCADREAC procedure for a product authorized in EU via MRP offers two different variants, which can be used to apply for a MA. In the following these two different variants are described. [7,32]

Description of the procedure for getting a MA - Variant I - after finalization of MRP

For variant I of the simplified procedure the application for MA is submitted any time after completion of the respective MRP when an updated AR is available.

The documents which have to be submitted by the applicant for this variant I were already described in section "3.4.3 Dossier requirements".

Description of the procedure for getting a MA - Variant II – in parallel with MRP

For variant II, the MAA is submitted after the RMS issued the AR and before the finalization of the MRP.

Therefore it is advisable that the applicant consults the relevant nCADREAC DRA before the submission in order to clarify any open issues.

Due to the time point of submission of the MAA, for variant II less documents are necessary because some of the documents requested for variant I are not yet available for variant II (like updated AR including harmonized SPC, consolidated list of questions raised by CMSs and the consolidated response of the applicant, PSUR, VARs and AR for VARs).

The documents which have to be submitted by the applicant for this variant II are described in section "3.4.3. Dossier requirements".

In the two mentioned documents describing the nCADREAC procedure for products authorized in EU via CP or MRP[31,6,32,7] the legal background, requirements and timelines for the nCADREAC procedures are described.

3.5 ASEAN

3.5.1 General Information Regarding ASEAN

Another important factor which should be mentioned and discussed in detail is the ASEAN countries (please refer also to the section "2 Status as of today").[8]

The ASEAN was established on 8 August 1967 in Bangkok by the five original member countries (Indonesia, Malaysia, Philippines, Singapore and Thailand). Meanwhile five additional countries (Brunei Darussalam, Vietnam, Laos, Myanmar and Cambodia) joined ASEAN.

In 1999 a harmonization initiative was started among the 10 ASEAN countries. One aim of this harmonization should be to harmonize quality guidelines that are valid for all countries involved. Another focus lies in the technical co-operation. Therefore the ACCSQ PPWG was established. The objective of the ACCSQ PPWG is the development of *"harmonization schemes of pharmaceuticals' regulations of the ASEAN member countries to complement and facilitate the objective of ASEAN Free Trade Area (AFTA), particularly, the elimination of technical barriers to trade posed by these regulations, without compromising on drug quality, safety and efficacy."* [8]

The strategy of the ACCSQ PPWG is the *"exchange of information on the existing pharmaceutical requirements and regulation implemented by each ASEAN member countries, to study the harmonized procedures and regulatory systems implemented in the ICH region, development of common technical dossiers with a view of arriving at MRAs (Mutual Recognition Arrangements)."* [8]

From August 2003 – December 2004 each ASEAN country should implement a trial implementation period for the ASEAN requirements (like ATCD and ACTR). The full implementation of the ASEAN requirements was originally planned for January 1st, 2005. The transition period for the ASEAN requirements was extended to December 31st, 2008 as it was not possible for the ASEAN countries to implement the ACTD until January 1st, 2005.

The full implementation of ACTD for new products was planned to be done in the ASEAN countries at different points in time between 2005 and 2008, which are summarized attached:

- Singapore and Malaysia by December 2005
- Thailand by December 2006
- Indonesia and Vietnam by December 2007
- Philippines, Cambodia, Laos and Brunei by December 2008.

As the full implementation of the ASEAN requirements (like ACTD and ACTR) in the ASEAN countries is not yet finalized, a prolongation/transition period was done. There is an interim period agreed wherein ACTD and national formats allowed in most of the ASEAN countries, whereas in some countries like Singapore ICH CTD is accepted.

The full implementation of ACTD for new products was expected by 31 December 2008 whereas the full implementation for currently registered products is expected to be done until 01 January 2012. According to information received from the ASEAN countries (January 2009) some of the ASEAN countries still accept the CTD-format for MAAs of NCEs and NBEs whereas for RENs and VARs only the ACTD-format is accepted by ASEAN countries. According to the information of the "forum institute seminar on October 21st and 22nd in Cologne" the full implementation of ACTD becomes mandatory by end of 2008 for MAAs and already registered products have to be transferred to ACTD until 2012.

All regulatory agencies in these 10 countries have a relatively weak infrastructure and limited resources. The agencies are structured differently and standards of scientific guidelines are not well established. A big problem of the agencies is the lack of consistency and the lack of transparency especially regarding the evaluation of dossier. To solve these problems they are constantly improving with more dialogues with the industry.

In all ASEAN countries a Certificate of a Pharmaceutical Product (CPP) from the reference country is required and builds the basis of the drug approval as the DRAs don't have the possibilities, capacities and scientific know-how to make a full evaluation of the submitted dossier (especially with regard to preclinical and clinical data).

3.5.2 Dossier Format – ASEAN CTD

As mentioned before the ASEAN countries established the ACTD as their format for submissions. It is a standard derived from the ICH CTD. The ASEAN CTD is a guideline of the agreed upon common format for the preparation of a well-structured ACTD application that will be submitted to ASEAN regulatory authorities for the registration of pharmaceuticals for human use.[33]

The ACTD is similar to the ICH CTD. The ICH CTD is divided into 5 modules whereas the ACTD contains of 4 parts. The reason for doing this is the fact that the ASEAN countries normally receive a reference application, which is a dossier which was already approved in other countries in the world (mostly EU and USA) and make the evaluation of the parts mainly based on the overviews and summaries.

Based on this, the need for detailed documentation is in most of the ASEAN countries less compared to the ICH countries, e.g. most study reports are not required to be submitted.

The Module 1 of the CTD containing the regional registration and administrative information is still presented as Part 1 of the ACTD.

The Module 2 of the CTD does not exist itself for the ACTD. The Quality Overall Summary (QOS) and the overview and summaries of the nonclinical and clinical documentation (similar like the documents in ICH Module 2) are included at the beginning of these Parts. Part II of the ACTD contains the pharmaceutical-chemical-biological documentation (the quality information), which corresponds to the ICH Module 3. The nonclinical information is presented as Part III of the ACTD (equivalent to ICH Module 4) and the clinical documentation is contained in Part IV of the ACTD (to be consistent with ICH Module 5).

The differences between ICH-CTD[34] and ACTD[35] are presented in the attached comparison pyramid:

---

[33] *The ASEAN Common Technical Document (ACTD) for the registration of pharmaceuticals for human use – organization of the dossier*
http://www.hsa.gov.sg/publish/etc/medialib/hsa_library/health_products_regulation/western_me dicines/files_guidelines.Par.22449.File.dat/ACTD_OrganizationofDossier.pdf
[34] http://upload.wikimedia.org/wikipedia/en/a/a9/CTD_Pyramid.jpg - dated 27.04.2009
http://www.ectdblog.com/2008_05_01_archive.html
[35] http://www.ectdblog.com/2008_05_01_archive.html
http://1.bp.blogspot.com/_Yjwi3JtqDOY/SERNIifkrEI/AAAAAAAAKsQ/Zr22IcsU1R8/s1600-h/actd.png

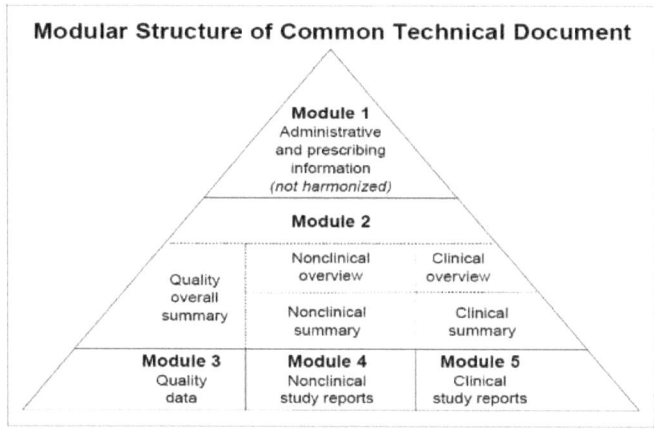

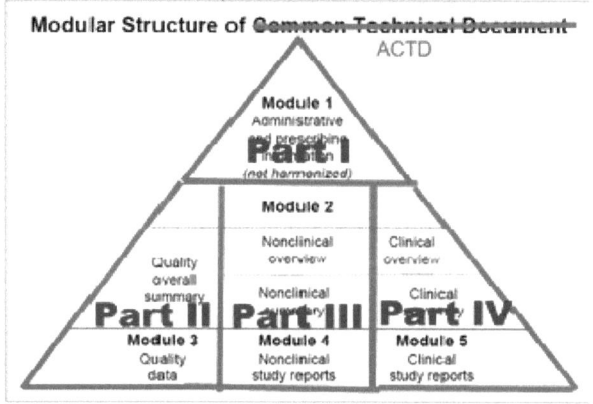

As demonstrated above the ACTD is organized in four parts[33]:

- Part I: ToC, Administrative Data and Product Information
- Part II: Quality Document
- Part III: Nonclinical Document
- Part IV: Clinical Document

The details of the different parts of ACTD are provided in appendix 9 ("APPENDIX 9: Table of Contents for ACTD").

3.5.3 Dossier Requirements

The requirements for the dossier for the ASEAN countries are in principle very similar to the requirements for the ICH countries. For ASEAN a guideline exists where the quality requirements for a MAA for an NBE and an NCE are described.[36] The detailed information of the dossier requirements for ASEAN countries is provided in APPENDIX 10 ("Dossier requirements for quality part of the dossier for ASEAN countries").
Additionally there are similar guidelines for the nonclinical[37] and clinical documentation.[38] As the guidelines are in principle very similar to the ICH CTD regulations, they will not be described here again in details.
The only important thing is to remember that the nonclinical overview and summary as well as the clinical overview and summary is put at the beginning of part 3 and 4 followed then by the study reports and literature. For some ASEAN countries these nonclinical and clinical overviews and summaries are sufficient and no additional study reports need to be submitted. In most cases it is sufficient to submit some publications from the mentioned studies in addition to the nonclinical and clinical overviews and summaries.
But for the full evaluation (which means a complete evaluation of the MAA dossier) in Singapore it is mandatory to submit the whole data package (full CMC, full nonclinical and full clinical data package). So far Health Sciences Authority (HSA) also accepts the ICH CTD dossier for MAAs although it would be appreciated to submit the dossier in ACTD format.
Additionally in Singapore there are additional requirements existing besides the ACTD and ACTR requirements. In Singapore there are some specific documents requested from the HSA like the preparation for a specific QOS.

---

[36] *The ASEAN Common Technical Dossier (ACTD) for the registration of pharmaceuticals for human use – Part II Quality*
http://www.hsa.gov.sg/publish/etc/medialib/hsa_library/health_products_regulation/western_me dicines/files_guielines.Par.28201.File.dat/ACTD_PartIIQuality_Apr05.pdf
http://www.hsa.gov.sg/publish/hsaportal/en/health_products_regulation/western_medicines/guid elines.html

[37] *The ASEAN Common Technical Dossier (ACTD) for the registration of pharmaceuticals for human use – Part III Nonclinical document*
http://www.hsa.gov.sg/publish/hsaportal/en/health_products_regulation/western_medicines/guid elines.html
http://www.hsa.gov.sg/publish/etc/medialib/hsa_library/health_products_regulation/western_me dicines/files_guidelines.Par.59468.File.dat/ACTD_PartIIINonClinical_Nov05.pdf

[38] *The ASEAN Common Technical Dossier (ACTD) for the registration of pharmaceuticals for human use – Part IV Clinical document*
http://www.hsa.gov.sg/publish/hsaportal/en/health_products_regulation/western_medicines/guid elines.html
http://www.hsa.gov.sg/publish/etc/medialib/hsa_library/health_products_regulation/western_me dicines/files_guidelines.Par.54671.File.dat/ACTD_PartIVClinical_Nov05.pdf

Within the "Guidance on medicinal product registration in Singapore"[39] the dossier requirements for the dossier for MAAs are described.

Within this guidance document the preparation of the QOS for NCEs (described in APPENDIX 8 of the guideline) and QOS for NBEs (described in APPENDIX 9 of the guideline) is described.[39]

The QOS for NCEs should be presented as a summary of the quality part (CMC part) of the NDA.[36] It is requested to submit a hard copy as well as an electronic copy for review. In principle the content of the QOS for NCEs is very similar to the QOS for the ICH dossier. There is some additional information requested like indicating for each section the "hard copy location/pages and e-copy location/file number".

Additionally the applicant has to fill out a tick box for Drug Substance (DS) general information.[39]

"For NCEs the following information are requested:

Check appropriate tick box
☐	DMF (open) is attached
☐	DMF (open and restricted) and Letter of Access to be submitted by DDMMYYYY (within month of Pharmaceutical Regulatory and Information Systems (PRISM) submission) or Letter of Access to the DMF filed with HAS (015:_____) is provided
☐	CEP (Certificate of suitability from European Directorate for the Quality of Medicines & HealthCare (EDQM)) for DS is attached. CEP number:
☐	CEP for raw materials and excipients is attached
☐	DS meets the current Pharmacopoeia of the United States (USP)/ European Pharmacopoeia (Ph.Eur.)/Japanese Pharmacopoeia (JPh) (delete as appropriate) requirements
☐	DS meets other pharmacopoeia standards
☐	DS meets in-house specifications
☐	DS meets other pharmacopoeia standards. Analytical methods and appropriate analytical method validation data are included in the dossier.
☐	DS meets in-house specifications. Analytical methods and appropriate analytical method validation data are included in the dossier.

---

[39] *Guidance on Medicinal Product Registration in Singapore (effective January 1, 2009)*
http://www.hsa.gov.sg/publish/hsaportal/en/health_products_regulation/western_medicines/guidelines.html
http://www.hsa.gov.sg/publish/etc/medialib/hsa_library/health_products_regulation/western_medicines/files_guidelines.Par.15295.File.dat/Guidance%20on%20Medicinal%20Product%20Registration%20in%20Singapore%202009_Complete%20with%20Appendices.pdf

Whereas for NBEs the table looks like this:

Check appropriate tick box	
☐	CEP for raw materials and excipients is attached
☐	Plasma Master file (PMF)
☐	Site Master File (SMF)
☐	DS meets in-house specifications. Analytical methods and appropriate analytical method validation data are included in the dossier."

There are also some recommendations how specifications, validation of analytical methods or batch analyzes should be presented.

In principle the QOS prepared for the ICH countries can be used also for Singapore. In some special cases it might be necessary to add some tables specifically requested for Singapore. But it can be discussed with HSA in most cases whether additional work is really needed as in principle the information requested are identical to the QOS for ICH countries.

3.5.4 Registration Procedures

The different registration procedure for ASEAN countries will be described on the example of Singapore. Singapore is one of the founder countries of ASEAN and is one of the leading countries within ASEAN.

On the homepage of the HSA[40] they described their responsibilities and functions:

"The Therapeutic Products Division (TPD) is responsible for the registration of medicines and the continual review of approved medicinal products. TPD will facilitate the timely introduction and availability of new and innovative quality medicines in Singapore and the region, including medicines targeted for diseases prevalent in the region.

The main activities relating to the control of medicinal products include:

- *Evaluation and approval of applications for new product licenses, amendment and REN of existing product licenses, as well as the continual review of registered medicinal products.*

- *Evaluation and approval for import of unregistered medicinal products on a named patient basis.*

---

[40] *Homepage of Health Sciences Authority – health products regulations - medicines:*
http://www.hsa.gov.sg/publish/hsaportal/en/health_products_regulation/western_medicines.html

- *Approval for the import of medicinal products for the purpose of re-export.*
- *Evaluation and approval of applications for licenses for the purpose of importation of registered medicinal products on a per consignment basis.*
- *Evaluation, approval and monitoring of clinical trials on medicinal products.*
- *Secretariat support for the Medicines Advisory Committee (MAC) and the Medical Clinical Research Committee (MCRC)."*

In Singapore exists in principle 3 types of registration procedures: [39]

- Full evaluation route
- Abridged evaluation route
- Verification route

Before submission of the MAA for an NBE or NCE the applicant should check which type of procedure is applicable for the MAA of the medicinal product ("pre-submission consultation").

The full evaluation route is applicable if no DRA has granted the MA for the medicinal product before.

The abridged evaluation route applies to MAAs of NCEs or NBEs if at least one DRA has approved the medicinal product before submission of the dossier in Singapore.

The verification route can only be used if the medicinal product is already approved by two HSA reference DRAs (so called benchmarked DRAs) (US (FDA), EU (EMA), AUS (Therapeutic Goods Administration (TGA)), United Kingdom (UK) (Medicines and Healthcare products Regulatory Agency (MHRA)) and Canada (Health Canada)) and if ARs from these two DRAs are available. This procedure is only possible for NCEs, not for NBEs due to the complexity of NBEs.

3.5.4.1 Full Evaluation Route

The full evaluation route is applicable for MAAs of NCEs and NBEs if no other DRA has approved the medicinal product as defined by World Health Organization (WHO) at the time of submission.

Using this evaluation route the Therapeutic Products Division (TPD) will provide first evaluation and approval of the dossier in the world for a new innovative product which has not received any authorization by any other DRA worldwide. This evaluation time takes 270 working days.

This route is applicable for innovative products containing an NBE or NCE (NDA-1) or a registered chemical or biological entity used in a new dosage form, new combination of registered chemical/biological entities (NDA-2) or subsequent strengths of innovative products (NDA-3).[39]

The ICH CTD as well as the ACTD are accepted submission formats for the MAA using the full evaluation route.

The applicant should inform HSA at least two months before submission about the intended submission date.

As the HSA will perform a complete evaluation of the dossier it is necessary to provide them with a complete CTD dossier. Full information on chemical/biological development, pharmaceutical/genetic development, toxicological and pharmacological data and clinical data must be submitted to support the MAA. For the quality part of the dossier all information regarding DS and Drug Product (DP) need to be submitted. For nonclinical part the complete dossier including all pharmacological, pharmacokinetic and toxicological data must be submitted. All documentation (including all study reports from Phase I, II and III with tables and appendices) has to be submitted for the clinical part of dossier.

3.5.4.2 Abridged Evaluation Route

The abridged evaluation route applies for MAAs of NCEs or NBEs if at least one DRA has approved the medicinal product before submission of the dossier in Singapore. All facts regarding product quality and direction of use (including dosing regimen(s), indication(s) and patient group(s)) should be the same as approved by the competent DRA in the reference country.

For the abridged evaluation route the HSA will perform only an abridged evaluation of the dossier. This abridged evaluation of dossier takes 180 working days.

The technical dossier requires the complete quality part (CMC documentation) for DS and DP and the nonclinical overview. For clinical data package the clinical overview, summaries of clinical efficacy and clinical safety, synopsis of relevant studies (mainly Phase II and III), a tabular listing of the clinical development program and study reports of pivotal studies are requested (the tables and appendices of the pivotal study reports can be submitted upon request of HSA).[39]

In case of a life-saving drug the applicant can ask for priority review if there is unmet medical need.

The following aspects are considered for acceptance for priority review: [39]

- Drug is intended for a life threatening disease/condition and demonstrate potential to address a local unmet medical need

Unmet medical need is defined by: [39]

- Absence of treatment options

- Lack of save and effective alternatives and the drug would be a significant improvement compared to available alternatives, as demonstrated by

  - Evidence of increased efficacy in treatment, prevention or diagnosis or

  - Elimination/reduction of treatment-limiting adverse drug reactions

Local public health concerns which may lead to priority review are the following diseases:

- Cancers

- Infectious diseases: dengue, tuberculosis, hepatitis, malaria

The justification why the application should be considered for priority review should be submitted together with the request for priority review. The justification should contain information how the product is expected to benefit for patients by: [39]

- How serious is the disease?

  - Seriousness of the disease condition, local & worldwide morality rates, anticipated morbidity and defibrillation as consequence of the disease

- What is the clinical relevance in the local population?

  - Local epidemiology data & requests trough "named –patient" exemptions

- Is there evidence for unmet medical need?

  - Unmet needs, available treatment options and inadequacy of available therapies

- How is the drug going to address the identified unmet medical need?
  - Extend to which the product is expected to have a major impact on medical practice, its major benefit, and unmet medical needs can be addressed
- What is the scientific basis?
  - The strength of evidence supporting the claims of addressing unmet medical needs, or, of significant improvements compared to available treatment

The written request for priority request with justification has to be submitted at the time point of filing the application. The applicant will be informed of the outcome at the point of acceptance of application after screening. HSA has also the right to reject the request for priority review if is considered appropriate.[39]

3.5.4.3 Verification Route

The verification route can only be used if the medicinal product is already approved by two benchmarked DRAs (so called reference authorities) and if ARs from these two DRAs are available. These benchmarked DRAs or reference authorities are FDA (US), EMA (EU), TGA (AUS), MHRA (UK) and Health Canada (Canada).

The applicant has to decide and declare which of the two reference authorities is the primary reference agency because all facts regarding product quality and direction of use (including dosing regimen(s), indication(s) and patient group(s)) should be the same as approved by the chosen primary reference agency. The verification route dossier has to be submitted at least 3 years from the date of approval by the chosen primary reference authority. The primary reference authority is defined as the reference authority for which qualifying supporting documents, as outlined in the "Guidance on medicinal product registration in Singapore" will be submitted by the applicant.[39]

The assessment using the verification route is based on the full ARs of the reference DRAs. Therefore the complete quality and clinical ARs are requested to enable the effective verification process. The ARs should also include all annexes and all questions & answers. The quality part of the dossier (pharmaceutical-chemical-biological documentation (QOS and ICH Module 3)) should include the initial submitted dossier to the primary reference authority, all questions and answers between primary reference authority and applicant (answers should be accompanied by the supporting documentation used in responses of questions) as well as all reports and/or documentation pertaining to post-approval VARs approved by the primary reference authority.[39] Additionally the nonclinical overview must be submitted. As clinical data package the clinical overview, summaries of clinical efficacy and clinical safety, synopsis of relevant studies (mainly Phase II and III), a tabular listing of the clinical development program and study reports of pivotal studies are requested (the tables and appendices of the pivotal study reports can be submitted upon request of HSA).[39] As mentioned before the complete ARs as well as other supporting documents from the primary reference agency are requested as tabulated below[39]:

Primary reference agency	Documentary requirements
AUS TGA	• Clinical and quality ARs, including all annexes, questions an answer documents between the applicant and the agency • Delegate's overview • Pre- Australian Drug Evaluation Committee (ADEC) response • ADEC minutes • ARs and/or documents pertaining to post-approval VARs, if applicable
Health Canada	• Clinical and quality ARs, including all annexes, questions an answer documents between the applicant and the agency • ARs and/or documents pertaining to post-approval VARs, if applicable
EMA	• Summary of CHMP opinion • European ARs (i.e. Rapporteur, CoRapporteur as well as the joint clinical and joint quality ARs), including all annexes, questions an answer documents between the applicant and the agency • ARs and/or documents pertaining to post-approval VARs, if applicable
UK MHRA	• Clinical and quality ARs, including all annexes, questions an answer documents between the applicant and the agency • ARs and/or documents pertaining to post-approval VARs, if applicable
US FDA	• Clinical and quality ARs (unredacted), including all annexes, questions an answer documents between the applicant and the agency • ARs and/or documents pertaining to post-approval VARs, if applicable

The ARs must be unredacted or unedited. Reports available from public domain are not acceptable.

Additionally, the following documents have to be submitted to HSA[39]:

- Official approval letter or an equivalent document from relevant primary reference agency that certifies the registration status of the DP
- GMP certificate for DP of the primary reference agency
- SPC/PIL currently approved by the primary reference agency
- *"Official letter declaring that the application as submitted to HSA or similar direction(s) of use, indication(s), dosing regimen(s) and/or patient group(s) have not been rejected, withdrawn, approved via appeal process or pending deferral by any competent DRA with reasons in each case if applicable*
- Official letter declaring that all aspects of the product's quality intended for sale in Singapore are *identical* as currently approved by the primary reference agency. This includes, but is not limited to, the formulation, site(s) of manufacture, release and shelf-life specifications, primary packaging and the PI/PIL. For example, if product was approved by FDA and EMA and the assessment report was from EMEA, the Singapore proposed product and PI/PIL should be identical to the currently approved EMEA product."

The data package submitted to HSA must be identical to the data package submitted to the reference authorities. Should there be differences between the dossier submitted to the HSA compared to the dossier submitted to reference authorities this will not delay the processing of the application by HSA but may lead to a switch of the dossier to an abridged evaluation route. The switch to an abridged evaluation route might be done if significant undisclosed differences between dossier submitted to HSA and reference authorities have been detected.

The verification route procedure is only possible for MAAs of NCEs, not for MAAs of NBEs due to the complexity of NBEs. The verification route takes only 60 working days.[39]

3.6 CHINA
3.6.1 Dossier Format

In China there is no special format required, therefore the ICH CTD can be used.

3.6.2 Dossier Requirements

The basis for the dossier requirements as well as the registration procedures in China are laid done in the "Drug Registration Regulation (SFDA Order 28)".[41]
There in the general principles, the basic requirements, clinical trials of drugs, application and approval of new drugs, generic drugs or imported drugs as well as applications for Over the Counter (OTC) drugs are described.
In Chapter 4 "Application and Approval of New Drugs" of this drug regulation the definition of new drugs are described in article 45: *"SFDA may use special approval process for the following new drug, where detail regulation will be promulgated separately:*

1. *New drug material and its preparation, active ingredients and its preparation extracted from plant, animal and minerals, which have not been marketed in China and;*
2. *chemical drug raw material and its preparations, and/or biological product that have not been marketed domestically or outside China;*
3. *New drugs for AIDS, cancer and orphan disease that are superior to the marketed drugs.*
4. *New drugs which treat diseases for which there is no effective therapy.*

For those drugs meeting the above provisions of this Regulation, during the drug registration, the applicant may apply for a special approval, SFDA shall organize specialist meeting to decide whether to use special approval for the drug application. Detailed provisions of special approval shall be promulgated separately."

The details regarding dossier requirements for NCEs are provided in annex 2 of the drug registration regulation "Registration Categories and Application Information Requirements of Chemical Drugs"[42] and for NBEs in annex 3 of the drug registration

---

[41] *Drug Registration Regulation (SFDA Order 28) (Translation by RDPAC, for Member use only) Drug Registration Regulation was approved on June 18, 2007 by SFDA executive meeting and is hereby published, which become effective from October 1, 2007. SFDA Commissioner, Shao Minli, July 10, 2007*
[42] *Annex 2: Registration Categories and Application Information Requirements of Chemical Drugs*

regulation "Registration Categories and Application Information Items Requirements of Biological Products".[43]

According the paragraph I "registration categories" of annex 2 of the drug registration regulation "Registration Categories and Application Information Requirements of Chemical Drugs"[42] the following registration categories are covered as NCEs:

1) *"New chemical entity never marketed in any country.*
   i. *Drug substance and its preparations made by synthesis or semi-synthesis.*
   ii. *Chemical monomer (including drug substance and preparation) extracted from natural sources or by fermentation.*
   iii. *Optical isomer (including drug substance and preparation) obtained by chiral separation or synthesis.*
   iv. *Drug with fewer components derived from marketed multi-component drug.*
   v. *New combination products.*
   vi. *A preparation already marketed in China but with a newly added indication not yet approved in any country.*
2) *Drug preparation with changed administration route and not marketed in any country*
3) *Drug marketed ex-China, including:*
   i. *Drug substance and its preparations, and / or with changed dose form, but no change of administration route.*
   ii. *Combination preparations, and / or with changed dose form, but no change of administration route.*
   iii. *Preparations with changed administration route and marketed ex-China.*
   iv. *A preparation already marketed in China but with a newly added indication approved ex-China.*
4) *Drug substance and its preparation with changed acid or alkaline radicals (or metallic elements), but without any pharmacological change, and the original drug entity already approved in China.*
5) *Drug preparation with changed dose form, but no change of administration route, and the original preparation already approved in China,*
6) *Drug substance or preparation following national standard."*

---

[43] *Annex 3: Registration Categories and Application Information Items Requirements of Biological Products*

The documents which are requested for an MAA dossier of an NCE are described in paragraph II "Application dossier item" of annex 2 of the drug registration regulation "Registration Categories and Application Information Requirements of Chemical Drugs"[42] are divided to the following four parts:
a) Summary
b) Pharmaceutical data
c) Pharmacology and toxicology study information
d) Clinical Study Information

The detailed list of documents required within these four parts is provided in appendix 11 ("APPENDIX 11: Dossier requirements for an NCE in China").[42]
The dossier requirements in principle are quite similar to the requirements for ICH region, only the administrative part of the dossier where local documents are requested differs.
For further details the table of the application information items is provided in appendix 12 ("APPENDIX 12: Table of application information item for China").

The dossier requirements for NBEs are described in annex 3 "Registration Categories and Application Information Items Requirements of Biological Products"[43]. In paragraph 1 the different registration categories of NBEs are described:

1) *"Biological products not yet marketed at domestic or overseas.*
2) *Mono-Clonal Antibody*
3) *Gene therapy, somatic cell therapy as well as the preparations.*
4) *Allergen products.*
5) *Multi component products with bioactivity extracted from, or by fermentation from human and / or animal tissues and / or body fluid,*
6) *New combination product made from the already marketed biological products.*
7) *A product that is marketed already overseas but not yet marketed domestic.*
8) *Some of the strains used for preparing of micro-ecological products not yet approved.*
9) *Products with not completely same structure with the already marketed products and not yet marketed at domestic or overseas (including Amino Acid Locus Mutation / Absence, modification caused by a different expression system, deletion, changed interpretation, as well as chemical modifications of the product).*
10) *Products with a method of preparation different with the already marketed one, (such as use of different expression system, host cells).*

11) Products first time made with DNA recombination technology (such as use of recombination technology to replace the synthesis technology, tissue extraction or fermentation technology).
12) Products transformed from non-injection into injection, or topical use into systemic use, and not yet marketed at domestic or overseas.
13) The marketed products with a change in dosage form but no change in route of administration.
14) Products with a change in route of administration (excluding the above Category 12).
15) Biological products admitted with National Standards."

The documents which are requested for an MAA dossier of an NBE are described in paragraph II "Application dossier item" of annex 3 of the drug registration regulation annex 3 "Registration Categories and Application Information Items Requirements of Biological Products"[41],[43] are divided to the following five parts:
a) Summary information
b) Pharmaceutical Study Information
c) Pharmacology and Toxicology Study Information
d) Clinical Study Information
e) Others

The detailed list of documents required within these five parts is provided in appendix 13 ("APPENDIX 13: Dossier requirements for an NBE in China").

As for the NCE the dossier requirements in principle are quite similar to the requirements for ICH region, only the administrative part of the dossier where local documents are requested differs.

For further details the table of the requirement of application information is provided in appendix 14 ("APPENDIX 14: Table of application information items for China").
Since November 2009 China is classified as climatic zone IVB which needs to be taken into consideration regarding the stability data needed for a new MAA.

3.6.3 Registration Procedures

According to the current information there are two different registration procedures available in China.

On the one hand there is the standard review procedure which is applicable for most of the NDAs. The review time for an NDA for an NCE takes approx. 13.5 months whereas the NDA for an NBE takes approx. 24 months. During the standard review procedure it is not possible to have any consultation of CDE in order to discuss topics of the NDA procedure. Also rolling submission of the NDA dossier is not possible for the standard review procedure.

The second registration procedure which is established by SFDA as of January 1st, 2009 is the special review procedure. This new procedure is applicable for NCEs or NBEs which are not yet approved in any market, for new medicinal products which are used for treatment of AIDS, malignant tumor and/or rare disease and have obvious clinical therapeutically advantages and for new medicinal products which treat diseases for which there is no effective therapy. The review time for an NDA under this special review procedure takes approx. 12 months. Another advantage of the special review procedure is that a rolling submission is permitted (e.g. safety, stability, CMC development, etc.) and also pre- and in-process consultation at CDE during the NDA review process is allowed. The advantage of special review procedure will be lost once the drug is approved in any country worldwide.

Please find enclosed a summary table comparing the two different review procedures:

	Standard Review Procedure	Special Review Procedure (SFDA issued in Jan. 2009)
Scope	Most applications go through this Standard Review Procedure	1. NCE or new bio-product which are not yet approved in any market 2. New drugs which are used for treatment of AIDS, malignant tumor and/or rare disease and have obvious clinical therapeutically advantages 3. New drugs which treat diseases for which there is no effective therapy
Timeline (Chemical Drugs)	IND: 10.5 months NDA: 13.5 months	IND/Clinical Trial Application (CTA): 8 – 9 months NDA: 12 months
Rolling Submission	Not allowed	Allowed (e.g. safety, stability, CMC development, etc.)
CDE Consultation	No	Pre- & In-process consultation is permitted

3.7 BRAZIL

3.7.1 Dossier Format

The format and content of an MAA of a medicinal product, which is called Product Registration Dossier (PRD) in Brazil is defined by the type of product.

There exists respective format and content regulations for the following categories of medicinal products:

- New products
- Similar products
- Generic products
- Herbal medicinal products
- Biological and blood products
- Allergenic products
- Specific medicinal products
- Medicinal products exempt from registration
- Dynamized medicinal products

The following product types are regarded as biological product and have to comply with the guidelines in Resolution RDC 315 of 26-Oct-2005[44]:

- Vaccines
- Hyperimmune serums
- Blood by products
- Biomedicines (products obtained from biological fluids or animal tissues and obtained by biotechnological processes)
- Probiotics
- Biological products formulated with live; attenuated or inactivated microorganisms
- MAbs
- Allergens

---

[44] *Resolution RDC 315 of 26-Oct-2005 - Brazilian Official Gazette of 10/31/05*

Antibiotics and conjugated estrogens are not regarded as biological products.

For this dissertation only the types "new products" and "biological products" are relevant and the regulatory requirements for these two types of products were analyzed.

There is no special format like the CTD-format (ICH-countries), the ACTD (ASEAN countries) or Medicines Registration Form (MRF) (South Africa) for providing the PRD to the Brazilian Health Surveillance Agency (ANVISA). It is only important that the whole documentation which is required is contained in the PRD and that all documentation is in Portuguese.

For most types of medicinal products (i.e. NBEs and NCEs) the PRD should contain: Administrative documents:

- Petition formularies

- Receipt of the payment of the respective fee

- Copy of the operating license

- Copy of the inscription of the responsible professional at the professional council

- Copy of the dossier notification protocol of the pilot batches manufacturing

- GMP Certificate issued by the ANVISA or copy of the protocol of the inspection request

- Copy of the operating authorization and of the special operating authorization, if applicable

Technical documents, including:

- Manufacturing and quality control (QC)

- Labeling

- Clinical and non-clinical studies (when applicable)

In December 2009 new requirements regarding labeling documentation (RDC 47-2009[45]) were published which need to be taken into consideration for a new MAA.

Detailed information which is required for NBEs and NCEs are described in the next section (section 3.7.2 Dossier requirements).

---

[45] *Resolution RDC 47 – 2009 of 08 September 2009 - Novas Regras para Bulas de Medicamentos*

3.7.2 Dossier Requirements

According to the Brazilian law (Resolution RDC 136 of 29-May-2003[46]) a product is regarded as a new product if the product is not yet approved for marketing in Brazil by Brazilian Health Surveillance Agency (ANVISA).

The resolution RD 136[46] defines the following medicinal products as new medicinal products:

- A product containing a synthetic or semi-synthetic active pharmaceutical ingredient (API) (isolated or in association)

- New pharmaceutical forms, new strengths, new routes of administration and new therapeutic indications in Brazil, of a product containing a synthetic or semi-synthetic API. This product have to be developed by a pharmaceutical laboratory which is not MAH of products containing already the specific API

- A product that results from:
    - A modification of the pharmacokinetic properties
    - Withdrawal of an API of a product already registered at the ANVISA
    - New salts, isomers, although the corresponding molecular entity has been already approved for registration

- Reference products: A reference product is defined as the innovator product which is a new product approved for marketing in Brazil and on which generic applications can make reference to. For this innovator product the efficacy and the

- Safety were proven by appropriate scientific studies approved for marketing in Brazil[47,48].

The dossier requirements for biological products are slightly different than for other new medicinal products.

---

[46] *RESOLUTION - RDC N° 136 OF MAY 29, 2003 - UNION OFFICIAL GAZETTE OF 02/06/2003*
[47] *Law 9.787 of 10-Feb-1999 - Brasília, February 10th 1999, 178th of the Independence and 111st of the Republic - FERNANDO HENRIQUE CARDOSO; José Serra*
[48] *Decree 3.961 of 10-Oct-2001*

The dossier requirements for a new medicinal product in Brazil are quite similar than in other countries. Nevertheless there are also some differences compared to e.g. EU, like requesting manufacturing batch records for DP, stability data for 30°C/75% rh for long term stability and the mandatory request for Phase III clinical data independent of the clinical indication.

Based on the Brazilian regulations and experiences some administrative documents (like CPP, Power of Attorney, GMP certificates, manufacturing authorizations, Authorization for the use of trademark) are required for new medicinal products which are imported to Brazil. The detailed list of administrative documents required are provided in appendix 15 ("APPENDIX 15: Administrative documents are required for new medicinal products which are imported to Brazil").

For the technical dossier (pharmaceutical/chemical/biological, preclinical and clinical documentation) there are in principle similar documents required than in the ICH region. A detailed list of required documents for NCEs and NBEs are provided in appendix 16 ("APPENDIX 16: Dossier Requirements (pharmaceutical/chemical/biological, preclinical and clinical documentation) for Brazil").

3.7.3 Registration Procedures

The applicant submits the registration dossier (PRD) to the ANVISA. The registration dossier contains of administrative documents, petition formularies, the technical report, the preclinical and clinical studies report and the price report. For products which are manufactured outside Brazil and have to be imported the applicant has to inform the ANVISA if the product will be imported as bulk product, in primary package or as final product. All documents have to be submitted in Portuguese. The official documents, which are CPP and GMP certificates, have to be certified and legal translated, besides a notary copy of the original.

Normal registration procedure

The PRD is submitted at the "Unidade de Atendimento e Protocolo" (UNIAP) (Services and Filing Unit) – subordinated to the Gerência Geral de Gestão Administrativa e Financeira, (General Office of Finance and Administration) of the ANVISA.[49]

---

[49] http://www.anvisa.gov.br- dated 22.07.2009

The medicinal product registration approval process is divided into three steps:[50]

- Step I: Filing
  - Preliminary documental analysis at the UNIAP
- Step II: Review
  - Analysis by the general office of drugs (Gerência-geral de Medicamentos) (GGMED)
- Step III: Approval
  - Publication of the Product Registration Approval in the Brazilian Official Gazette (Diário Oficial da Uniao) (DOU)

Step I: Filing
The PRD review process starts when the applicant fills out the petition formularies electronically at the ANVISA electronic system. These petition formularies go to the respective technical area of the ANVISA for a preliminary analysis until the complete application is submitted to UNIAP. [50]

Due to internal processes it might happen that the technical area starts with the revision of PRD first when the complete application was submitted and the PRD is complete.
After submission of the PRD to UNIAP the applicant receives a process number which is a reference number. This number serves to follow up the registration process and any other post-marketing application to be submitted for the medicinal product once it is already registered at the ANVISA. After receipt of the process number, the PRD is checked whether it complies with the list of documents required by the respective legislation (depending on type of product) by making a documental analysis. Should it be recognized that the documents are not in line with those documents requested, UNIAP adds an identification of "incomplete documentation". Then the process goes to the respective technical area to be revised.[51]
As soon as the application is sent to the technical area of the ANVISA for a preliminary analysis, the applicant can follow the whole review process at the ANVISA's website.[49] In case of incomplete applications these information are placed in a specific site location that applicants can easily find out about their status.[50]

---

[50] *Private information received from Susan Koepke, Regulatory Affairs Director – Latin America, Merck Serono*
[51] *Resolution RDC 314 of 09-Dec-2004)*

The applicant has to access the electronic submission at the ANVISA's website[49] to complete the process documentation. The applicant submits "complementation of documents" using the appropriate front page. If the "complementation of documents" is not performed on the ANVISA website by the applicant before the start of the process review, the application will be rejected. [50]

Additionally an application is rejected if the respective fees are not paid by the applicant or when the electronic petition number used by the applicant was already utilized for another procedure. [50]

Step II: Review
After finalization of step I (preliminary documental analysis by UNAIP), the MAA is forwarded to the ANVISA's General Offices Divisions or Units which are responsible for the review of this respective type of application.[50]

For the evaluation process of new medicinal products and biological the responsible division is Coordenação de Pesquisa, Ensaios Clínicos, Medicamentos Biológicos e Novos (New Medicinal Products, Biologicals, Research and Clinical Studies Division) (GPBEN). This division is divided into several units. For biological products the review procedure is performed by the Coordenação de Produtos Biológicos e Hemoterápicos (Hemotherapic and Biologic Medicinal Products Coordination) (CPBIH) and for synthetic medicinal products the evaluation is performed by Coordenação de Medicamentos Sintéticos e Semi-Sintéticos (Synthetic and Semi- Synthetic Medicinal Products Coordination) (COMSI).

ANVISA may request additional data or information during the evaluation process of the application. Based on the outcome of the review process the approval is granted or not and the results are published at the DOU. [50]

The review of the PRD for new medicinal products is applicable for any new medicinal product application including herbal medicinal products, blood products and products subject to special control (narcotics and related substances).

The review process consists of the following steps: [50]

The administrative and the technical documents are checked by the GPBEN reviewer. In parallel the nonclinical and clinical documentation is sent to ad hoc consultants. They will review the nonclinical and clinical documentation and will prepare an expert report with a recommendation whether the medicinal product can be approved or not. Today the CATEME (Câmara Técnica de Medicamentos), the technical board for medicinal products, which previously discussed the PDR, evaluates only overall aspects related to medicinal products.

The final decision concerning the granting of a MA is made by the GPBEN. [50]

In case the new medicinal product is a biological product there are some differences between the review process compared to the above described process. [50]

For biological products the CPBIH is the responsible unit for checking the administrative and technical documentation and the information available regarding the product and/or manufacturers. Based on their review CPBIH decides whether a QC analysis of three batches has to be performed at the QC laboratory. The documents for these three batches are part of the PRD. If the CPBIH comes to the conclusion that the product has to undergo the QC analysis they will ask the applicant to send the respective samples to the "Instituto National de Controle de Qualidade em Saúde" (National institute of quality control and health) (INCQS). The INCQS is a unit of the Fundação Oswaldo Cruz (Oswaldo Cruz Foundation (FIOCRUZ)), which is linked to the Ministry of Health (MoH) with the goal to implement actions in the scientific and health technology areas. [50]

If the applicant has no samples of the required batches available he has to inform the CPBIH and INCQS accordingly and has to provide samples and documentation of three other batches. The samples accompanied by the respective documentation have to be provided to INCQS within 30 days. The applicant can apply for an extension of the deadline (up to two periods) in written format. In case the samples are not provided to INCQS within the timeline the application is regarded as rejected. [50]

The review of the quality part of a biological medicinal product application is also within the responsibility of INCQS. During the review of the quality party INCQS may request additional documents or information from the applicant. In case a request from INCQS arrives, the applicant has 30 days to answer the questions. Should an answer to the request not be possible within 30 days the applicant can apply for an extension of deadline (in total two extensions are possible). If the requests are not answered at all, the application will lead to an unapproved MA. [50]

During the general review process of the different divisions and units the applicant may receive requests for additional data/information in case an issue is not clear in the PRD and/or more information is needed. For answering such a request a 30 day period is planned. The applicant can apply for an extension of these 30 day period. The application for extension may be done by fax or by submitting a request to the ANVISA. During this "review process" (step II) the applicant can check the review status of his medicinal product on ANVISA's website section called "Consulta à Situação de Processos".[49] The applicant can ask for meetings with the respective technical staff member in charge of the applicant to discuss major issues. [50]

Step III: Approval
After finalization of the review process the GPBEN is responsible for the final decision relating to the application.
If the application is regarded as approvable, the MA will be granted which will be published in the DOU. Additionally ANVISA can provide a product registration certificate which is available for the applicant upon request. [50]
If the application is regarded as non-approvable, a publication of this refusal/ non-approval is made in the DOU. The applicant can apply for another review in case he can assess it appropriate. The decision for not approving a PRD of a medicinal product is mainly based on a lack of clinical data to support efficacy and safety and a lack of manufacturing and QC data to support quality of the final product. [50]

A typical publication in DOU of a PRD which was approved contains the following information:

- Name of the company
- Generic name of the product
- Trademark (brand name) of the product
- Therapeutic class
- Product registration number
- Marketing presentations
- Expiry period
- Process number (the one designated at the submission)
- Type of approval being granted: New product, Similar product and Generic product

The registration procedure for a new medicinal product (NCEs and NBEs) currently takes between 8 and 12 months. This is longer as originally described in the Law 6.360 of 23.09.1976.[52] Therein it is mentioned that the registration approval should be granted within a period of 90 days from the date of submission unless a request comes up during the review process. The formal review period which is established by ANVISA for a new biological product is 180 days. [50]

---

[52] *Law n° 6.360, of September 23, 1976 -*
OFFICIAL JOURNAL OF THE UNION OF SEPTEMBER 24, 1976 - Brasilia, September 23, 1976; 155 of Independence and 88 of the Republic. - Ernesto Geisel,
Paulo de Almeida Machadohttp://www.anvisa.gov.br/hotsite/genericos/legis/leis/6360_e.htm

Procedure for priority review/accelerated approval

ANVISA established the priority review with the publication of the Resolution RDC 28 of 04.04.2007[53] modified by Resolution RDC 16 of 13.03.2008[54].

Conditions for priority review:

- When post registration review is essential to avoid a lack of medicinal products that is the only one in the Brazilian market with a specific API, association, strength or pharmaceutical form

- When post registration review is essential to avoid a lack of medicinal product for the Unified Health System (SUS)

- When post registration applications refer to fractioned market presentations as established by Decree 5775/2006[55]

- Post registration and registration of medicinal products directed to SUS programs including vaccines and exceptional medicinal products

- Registration of medicinal products used in the prophylaxis or treatment of orphan drug diseases (diseases which have no commercial value) or emergent and re-emerging diseases

Priority review procedure

The application has to be made electronically on ANVISA's internet site at Serviços/ Atendimento/ Arrecadação Eletrônicos/ Peticionamento Eletrônico. The applicant has to enter his login and password.
The applicant has additionally to fill in a specific form directly online at the website. Additionally the following documents have to be provided:

- Rationale to support the priority review request (informing the process submission number)

---

[53] *Resolution RDC 28 of 04.04.2007 - RESOLUÇÃO RDC No- 28, DE 4 DE ABRIL DE 2007 - Dispõe sobre a priorização da análise técnica de petições, no âmbito da Gerência- Geral de Medicamentos da ANVISA, cuja relevância pública se enquadre nos termos desta Resolução. - DIRCEU RAPOSO DE MELLO*

[54] *Resolution RDC 16 of 13.03.2008 - RESOLUÇÃO N° 16, DE 13 DE MARÇO DE 2008 Altera a Resolução - RDC n° 28, de 4 de abril de 2007, que dispõe sobre a priorização de análise técnica de petições no âmbito da Gerência Geral de Medicamentos da ANVISA - DIRCEU RAPOSO DE MELLO*

[55] *Decree 5775/2006 - DECRETO No- 5.775, DE 10 DE MAIO DE 2006*
Dispõe sobre o fracionamento de medicamentos, dá nova redação aos arts. 2o e 9o do Decreto no 74.170, de 10 de junho de 1974, e dá outras providências - Brasília, 10 de maio de 2006; 185o da Independência e 118o da República - LUIZ INÁCIO LULA DA SILVA, José Agenor Álvares da Silva

- The original fee payment receipt which will be generated during the electronic submission as release from payment and is automatically attached to the process during the electronic procedure

- Major documents which support the priority review request like official letters and links to regulatory authorities in other countries which support the recognition of the orphan drug status

- Inform the applicant's e-mail address

All these additional documents have to be submitted as pdf-documents.

The priority review is divided into different phases. First of all, the priority request application is reviewed by a Technical Committee of GGMED of the ANVISA which takes a mean time of 20 days. This technical committee of GGMED will check the compliance of the request according to Resolution-RDC-28/2007[53]. They will issue a report to the GGMED General Manager who will then send the application for priority review in case the criteria are fulfilled.

After ANVISA has received the "green light" for priority review from GGMED General Manager, they have 75 days period time for review the priority request applications concerning medicinal products. This time is only applicable if no query is written. As soon as a query is issued, the whole review will take longer than the 75 days.

The applicant can follow the review status at the homepage of ANVISA under: *http://www.anvisa.gov.br/servicos/consulta_documentos.htm.*[56]

---

[56] *http://www.anvisa.gov.br/servicos/consulta_documentos.htm - dated 22.07.2009*

4 Comparison of the Pharmaceutical Legislation and Regulatory Requirements for a Marketing Authorization Application of a New Biological Entity and a New Chemical Entity within the Different Countries and Regions

As already discussed during the analysis of the pharmaceutical legislation and regulatory requirements for NCEs and NBEs in the different regions and countries it is obvious that the requirements for an MAA dossier for an NBE or NCE are more or less similar or even identical between the different regions and countries. The basis for the requirements (content) for an MAA dossier of an NBE or NCE is certainly set and developed by ICH. Based on the ICH requirements, a lot of non-ICH-countries adapt their requirements what have to be contained in an MAA dossier for an NBE or NCE to the ICH requirements (please refer to NtA Vol. 2).

The CTD format which was developed in order to have one global format for submissions in the ICH region is also used and accepted in quite a lot of non-ICH-countries.

In some non-ICH-countries there are no special requirements on a dossier format. They accept every dossier format as long as the required documents are contained in the dossier (examples are countries in LA like Argentina, Colombia or Brazil). Nevertheless, there are also countries which have their own format and request to submit the dossiers in their special format. Examples for these are e.g. South Africa, which uses the so-called MRF or the ASEAN countries which even developed their own ACTD format.

Countries which are very "near" to the EU (mainly countries in SEE) or even have the intention to become EU MS in the future have implemented the EU guidelines, regulations and requirements in their national law. Countries like Serbia or the CADREAC country Croatia therefore request the original EU dossier.

Based on experiences during the last years it can be said that a lot of non-ICH-countries have very similar requirements as the EU.
If the EU dossier for an MAA of an NBE or NCE is submitted in non-ICH-countries the chance is very high to obtain approval.

Nevertheless, there is on the other hand a quite high risk to submit the EU dossier in the non-ICH-countries due to confidentiality and IP issues. One issue in the non-ICH-countries is the fact that the applicant is often not absolutely sure whether the dossier submitted is kept confidential and never knows who might receive the dossier or a copy of the dossier. The risk is especially very high in countries where no patent protection or dossier protection is available and where a very strong generic industry, mainly local generic industry, is located.

This risk is especially applicable for the pharmaceutical-chemical-biological part of the dossier, i.e. Module 2.3 QOS and Module 3. The differences between dossier and dossier requirements for NCEs and NBEs are mainly within the CMC part of the dossier. The main differences between NCEs and NBEs occur in the DS part and the appendices. For detailed information please refer to the attached table in appendix 3 ("APPENDIX 3: Differences NBE and NCE with regard to Module 2 and 3").[12] The NBE is defined not only by the molecule itself but also by the manufacturing process. Based on this, the requirements on the CMC documentation which needs to be provided are higher and more complex than the documentation for NCEs.

Due to this confidentiality issue most of the companies submit in the non-ICH-countries a dossier - a so-called international dossier - with a reduced content especially regarding the CMC part where the highly confidential information is located. This is even more important for NBEs as within the CMC part the whole molecule, characterization and manufacturing process is described very detailed. It is advisable to reduce the CMC part for an MAA for an NBE and an NCE and to eliminate the highly confidential information in order to avoid that generic companies can easily copy the product.

Therefore as mentioned before a lot of companies create an international dossier which contains less information within the DS part and the appendices of the dossier. For an NBE especially the sections 3.2.S.2 (3.2.S.2.2 Description of Manufacturing Process and Process Controls, 3.2.S.2.3 Control of Materials, 3.2.S.2.5 Process Validation and/or Evaluation, 3.2.S.2.6 Manufacturing Process Development), 3.2.S.3. Characterization (3.2.S.3.1 Elucidation of Structure and other Characteristics) and 3.2.A.2 Adventitious Agents Safety Evaluation are often shortened and the highly confidential information is reduced or completely deleted. For the MAA dossier of an NCE it is also advisable to check whether some sections in the CMC part can be reduced in order to avoid providing highly confidential information to every authority within the world.

It is important that the non-ICH-countries receive the complete dossier which means that all sections of the ICH dossier should be contained even in the international dossier.

If an applicant just deletes some sections of the ICH dossier and submit an "incomplete" dossier the risk is very high that the authorities will ask for the missing sections. Therefore it is strongly recommended that only the content in some sections (especially in sections 3.2.S.2 and 3.2.S.3) should be reduced, so that there is a complete dossier only with reduced content submitted to the authority. This approach minimizes the hazard that the authorities recognize that some information are missing and will maybe not ask for additional information. One possibility to make these changes within the dossier is the creation of an MAA dossier for an NBE or NCE with the determination of a high granularity for documents in order to be able to exchange some documents or parts of documents quite easily for the international countries (e.g. in order to avoid to provide highly confidential information to these countries). This might reduce the workload for the people writing CMC documentation if high granularity documents are available (e.g. for each section and subsection one separate document is available), so that for the non-ICH countries only some documents can be used without making visual that a section or information is missing.

Countries within the non-ICH region where the EU dossier needs to be submitted are AUS, Croatia (as CADREAC country), Israel, South Africa, South Korea and CH. Based on my experiences in these countries there is no chance to submit only a reduced dossier as they will ask for the missing information. AUS, Croatia and CH are not seen as critical countries as they have some IP rights and patent protection laws in place. In countries like Israel, South Africa and South Korea there is the possibility to ask the authorities to sign a confidentiality agreement for the dossier submitted. This might be useful for some applicants even they cannot be 100% sure whether the authorities really keep the dossier confidential.

There are also some non-ICH-countries (like China, Taiwan, Mexico) which request more information and data for CMC part of the dossier as normally requested in the EU. China often requests more detailed information for NBEs (like details about the structure of the molecule, the vector (in case a vector is used), the manufacturing process or the characterization). Taiwan and Mexico request batch records for at least one batch which are normally not submitted to authorities as these are also confidential information. Mexico also requests some additional raw data (batch records of three batches for each manufacturer combined with corresponding Certificates of Analysis (CoAs) for DS, DP as well as for the excipients and chromatograms) in order to check the dossier very accurate. Without submission of these information the dossier is seen as incomplete and will not be evaluated.

The main focus for most of the regions outside ICH is laid done in the CMC section of the dossier as this is their main field of expertise. Therefore it is highly recommended that the CMC section should be as complete and comprehensive as possible to avoid questions. Based on the experiences most of the questions from non-ICH-countries will come back for this section of the dossier whereas for nonclinical section normally no or only very few questions are raised. For the clinical part of the dossier it depends on the country whether they have experts on the field or not whether questions are raised. There are countries within non-ICH-countries like AUS, CH or Singapore which are very experienced and have a lot of experts for the clinical section. They will definitely raise also questions for the clinical section of the dossier.

As some non-ICH-countries do not have so many expertise in the nonclinical and clinical field it is very important for them to receive a CPP from a benchmarked country like USA, EU, JP, CH, AUS or Canada. The CPP proofs that a benchmarked country has accessed the dossier and has granted based on their scientific evaluation the MA for the medicinal product.

The requirements within the nonclinical section (Module 4) and clinical section (Module 5) of the dossier are mainly identical within the different countries and regions.

In some non-ICH-countries it is sufficient to submit the Module 2 documents as nonclinical and clinical information (i.e. nonclinical and clinical overview as well as nonclinical and clinical summary). Modules 4 and 5 are sometimes not requested (e.g. in some LA countries) or it is sufficient to submit publications of the studies presented in Module 4 and 5. The study reports presented in Modules 4 and 5 are often not requested for these countries. As mentioned for some non-ICH-countries it is important to receive some publications of the clinical studies. This proofs that the studies are finalized and that the results of the studies were presented to scientific community and were made published. This is for countries which do not have the expertise and man power to evaluate the clinical section of a dossier (all study reports) by themselves very important. Some countries will grant an approval for some indications only after the study results are published in a publication (e.g. Malaysia).

In the other non-ICH-countries (e.g. the benchmarked countries like AUS, Canada and CH as well as SEE, some Asian countries or LA countries) it is recommended to submit the identical documentation for nonclinical and clinical part as in the EU. For the LA countries some parts of the dossier or even the whole dossier needs to be submitted in Spanish (for nearly all LA countries) or in Portuguese (e.g. for Brazil) to the authorities.

Other difference between the requirements within the different countries and regions are with regard to Module 1 of the MAA dossier. Module 1 differs partly heavily dependent on the country or region. But some documents of Module 1 are required in nearly every country. An example for a document of Module 1 which is requested at least in all non-ICH-countries except AUS, Canada and CH are the CPP. Other administrative documents like GMP certificates of manufacturer or CoAs are also required in most of the countries, at least in non-ICH. Labeling documents (SPC, PIL, mock-ups) are requested in every country worldwide within Module 1. Some countries in the non-ICH-region do not have a differentiation between a SPC (labeling information for health care professionals) and a PIL (labeling document for patients). They only have combined information which is intended to be used by health care professionals as well as by patients. For the creation of such a labeling document it is important that all essential information for the health care professionals are included as well as the document is in an intelligible language for the patients.

To sum up the differences between the requirements between the different regions and countries are mainly focused on Module 1 requirements. The dossier itself (Modules 2 – 5) is nearly identical for all regions. As mentioned above an international dossier with reduced content of CMC information should be created to avoid difficulties regarding confidentiality and/or IP issues. For the nonclinical and clinical section it is often enough to provide the Module 2 documents to some non-ICH-countries. This should be checked with the country before providing the dossier. For the clinical section it is advisable to provide some publications in addition or instead of the full study reports to the non-ICH-countries.

Comparison of different registration procedures in the different countries and pro/con arguments for each procedure:

Country/Region	Procedure	Pro	Con
EU	National procedure	* might be useful for a medicinal product which is specifically intended only for one EU MS	* not possible if product shall be registered in more than one EU MS * not possible for products which fall under Regulation 726/2004
	MRP	* can be used for medicinal products which already have a MA in at least one EU MS * "recognition" procedure – RMS gives an opinion and CMS recognized it (no new evaluation of the dossier by CMS) * updated AR from RMS has to be prepared within 90 days of receipt of the valid application * each CMS has the obligation to recognize the MA granted by the RMS within a period of 90 days	* not possible for products which fall under Regulation 726/2004 * often not really a "recognition" procedure - CMS does not accept the recommendation of RMS * in total quite long registration time (from RMS until national MAs in CMS are granted) * quite long registration time for initial MA in RMS (210 days) * national phase in CMS takes sometimes a lot of time (several months) (depending on the country) * different MAHs in the different EU MS
	DCP	* procedure faster than MRP * the DCP is open for medicinal products which are not yet approved in any EU MS at the time of application	* for medicinal product with no MA in an EU MS the DCP can be used alternatively * often not really a "recognition" procedure - CMS does not accept the

Country/Region	Procedure	Pro	Con
		* submission of the MAA dossier is done to the RMS and the CMSs in parallel	recommendation of RMS * initial MA not issued by RMS alone
		* AR from RMS is prepared in consultation with the CMSs * this AR is the basis for the RMS and CMSs to agree the terms for the MA * RMS,CMS phase can be quite short (120 days)	* quite long registration time (210 days) if after phase I (120 days) no agreement is reached * sometimes long national phases (depending on the country) * different MAHs in the different EU MS
	CP	* scientific evaluation done by CHMP (in which representatives of each EU MS are in) * one scientific opinion valid for the EU and Norway, Iceland and Liechtenstein * one registration for EU and Norway, Liechtenstein and Iceland * is optional for other innovative new medicinal products * the MAAs have to be submitted directly to the EMA in London * identical MA with identical label throughout EU * only one MAH for all countries	* the CP is compulsory for medicinal products derived from biotechnology and for new active substances for certain therapeutic areas like acquired immune deficiency syndrome (AIDS), cancer or viral diseases * identical MA with identical label throughout EU * if the CHMP opinion is negative no registration in EU and European Economic Area (EEA) * long registration time (246 days without clock-stops) (210 days scientific evaluation, 36 days for the preparation of the annexes to the Commission Decision plus 30 days)

Country/Region	Procedure	Pro	Con
	Accelerated assessment procedure	* for medicinal products of major therapeutic interest, and procedures for obtaining temporary authorizations subject to certain annually reviewable conditions * request for accelerated assessment procedure is submitted to CHMP and CHMP decide about the acceptance for accelerated assessment procedure * scientific evaluation done by CHMP in 150 days	* cannot be used for all types of products * only for medicinal products of major therapeutic interest, and procedures for obtaining temporary authorizations subject to certain annually reviewable conditions * At any time during the MAA, the CHMP may decide to continue the assessment under standard CP timelines (210 days) and to withdraw the granting of the accelerated assessment procedure. This might happen in case the CHMP is the opinion that it is no longer appropriate to conduct an accelerated assessment
USA	Full application	* valid for all NDAs and BLAs * quite short review time (10 months (at least for 90 % of NDAs and BLAs))	* long review times (10% of BLAs and NDAs needs more review time then 10 months)
	Accelerated Approval	* applicable only for drugs or biologics products which provides meaningful therapeutic benefit...over existing treatments *applicable for the treatment of a serious or life-threatening disease * the procedure allows the approval based on clinical trials using "a	* cannot be used for all types of products * only applicable for serious or life-threatening disease

100

Country/Region	Procedure	Pro	Con
		surrogate endpoint that is reasonable likely... to predict clinical benefit." instead of using standard outcome measures like survival or disease progression	
		* can be used for drugs for which the use could be considered safe and effective only under set restrictions which could include limited prescribing or dispensing	
	Priority Review	* can be used for medicinal products which are intended to address unmet medical need	* the priority review process starts only when a manufacturer officially submits an NDA/BLA
		* timing of the application (NDA/BLA) can be shortened from 10 months to 6 months	* does not have any influence on the timing or content of steps taken during the drug development or the testing of safety and efficacy
	Fast track mechanism	* is designed for certain products (product must concern a serious or life-threatening condition and has potential to address an unmet medical need)	* only applicable for serious or life-threatening disease which have potential to address unmet medical need
			* cannot be used for all types of products
		* close interaction with FDA – "discuss with FDA development plans and strategies before the official submission of the NDA/BLA"	* similar interactions to any sponsor who asks for FDA consultation throughout the development phases of a medicinal product
		* issues like elements of clinical study designs and	

101

Country/Region	Procedure	Pro	Con
		presentation whose absence at NDA/BLA can lead to a delay in approval decision of NDA/BLA could be clarified earlier with FDA	
		* shortening approval time (6 months instead of 10 months)	
		* opportunity of a rolling submission, i.e. to submit sections of an NDA/BLA to FDA as they are ready, rather than the standard requirement to submit a complete application at one time	
Croatia	National procedure	*only applicable for products which are authorized in EU via national procedure * not mandatorily the identical dossier as submitted in EU has to be submitted	* no real option as Croatian authority accept national procedure only for products which are authorized in EU via national procedure * complete evaluation of the dossier is done * a lot of questions especially for CMC expected as complete evaluation is done
	CADREA procedure MRP	* applicable for all products authorized in EU via MRP * CADREAC procedure can be done in parallel or after finalization of MRP * less or even no questions as Croatia recognized the EU procedure outcome * no complete	* identical dossier as submitted for MRP has to be submitted (confidentiality!)

Country/Region	Procedure	Pro	Con
		evaluation of dossier is done (ARs are therefore very important for evaluation)	
	CADREA procedure DCP	* applicable for all products authorized in EU via DCP * CADREAC procedure can be done in parallel or after finalization of DCP * less or even no questions as Croatia recognized the EU procedure outcome	* identical dossier as submitted for DCP has to be submitted (confidentiality!)
	CADREA procedure CP	* applicable for all products authorized in EU via CP * less or even no questions as Croatia recognized the EU procedure outcome	* identical dossier as submitted for CP has to be submitted (confidentiality!)
Singapore	Full evaluation route	* is applicable for MAAs of NCEs and NBEs if no other DRA has approved the medicinal product as defined by WHO at the time of submission * is applicable for innovative products containing an NBE or NCE (NDA-1) * ICH CTD as well as A-CTD dossiers are acceptable	* complete ICH dossier must be submitted for evaluation (confidentiality!) * long review time (270 working days)
	Abridged evaluation route	* applies for MAAs of NCEs or NBEs if at least one DRA has approved the medicinal product before submission of the dossier in Singapore * all facts regarding product quality and	* all facts regarding product quality and direction of use (including dosing regimen(s), indication(s) and patient group(s)) should be the same as approved by the competent DRA in the reference country

Country/Region	Procedure	Pro	Con
		direction of use (including dosing regimen(s), indication(s) and patient group(s)) should be the same as approved by the competent DRA in the reference country	
		* not complete ICH dossier is requested (regarding nonclinical less information are needed) (complete CMC part, nonclinical overview and clinical data package (clinical overview, summaries of clinical efficacy and clinical safety, synopsis of relevant studies (mainly Phase II and III), a tabular listing of the clinical development program and study reports of pivotal studies are requested))	* for CMC and clinical part of the dossier the complete documentation is requested
		* only abridged evaluation is performed	* only abridged evaluation is performed
		* this abridged evaluation of dossier which takes 180 working days	* this abridged evaluation of dossier which takes 180 working days
		* in case of a life-saving drug the applicant can ask for priority review if there is unmet medical need.	* no guarantee that HAS will accept the priority review for the life-saving drug
	Verification route	* can only be used if the medicinal product is already approved by two benchmarked DRAs (so called reference authorities) and if ARs from	* is only possible for MAAs of NCEs * is not possible for MAAs of NBEs due to the complexity of NBEs

Country/Region	Procedure	Pro	Con
		these two DRAs are available	
		* these benchmarked DRAs or reference authorities are FDA (US), EMA (EU), TGA (AUS), MHRA (UK) and Health Canada (Canada).	* the verification route dossier has to be submitted at least 3 years from the date of approval by the chosen primary reference authority
		* the assessment using the verification route is based on the full ARs of the reference DRAs. Therefore the complete quality and clinical ARs are requested to enable the effective verification process	* submission of all authority correspondence, Answers to Objections, ARs needed (confidentiality!)
		* very fast evaluation time (only 60 working days)	
China	Standard review procedure	* applicable for most of the NDAs	* long review times especially for NBEs (The review time for an NDA for an NCE takes approx. 13.5 months whereas the NDA for an NBE takes approx. 24 months)
			* no consultation of CDE in order to discuss topics of the NDA procedure possible during the procedure
			* rolling submission of the NDA dossier is not possible for the standard review procedure
	Special review procedure	* applicable for NCEs or NBEs under certain circumstances: • which are not yet approved in any market	* the advantage of special review procedure will be lost once the drug is approved in any country worldwide
			* usage in practical not really as China

105

Country/Region	Procedure	Pro	Con
		• for new medicinal products which are used for treatment of AIDS, malignant tumor and/or rare disease • have obvious clinical therapeutically advantages and for new medicinal products which treat diseases for which there is no effective therapy * the review time for an NDA under this special review procedure takes approx. 12 months * rolling submission is permitted (e.g. safety, stability, CMC development, etc.) * pre- and in-process consultation at CDE during the NDA review process is permitted	might normally not be the first country who issues the MA * review time only 1.5 months shorter than standard review procedure
Brazil	Normal registration procedure	* according to law the registration approval should be granted within a period of 90 days from the date of filing unless a request arises during the review process * the formal review period which is established by ANVISA for a new biological product is 180 days	* in practice the registration times are quite long (between 8 and 12 months) * the formal review period for NBE which is established by ANVISA is 180 days

106

Country/Region	Procedure	Pro	Con
	Procedure for priority review/accelerated approval	* short review time (75 or 90 days) but only if no inquiry is issued	* longer review time as soon as inquiry is issued * only applicable under very strict conditions (like medicinal products used in the prophylaxis or treatment of neglected diseases (orphan drugs) or emergent and re-emerging diseases)

Short evaluation of different registration procedures in different countries on the examples of EU, Croatia and China:

EU:
In EU it depends on the type of product which procedure can be used.

CP:
In the CP the MAA dossier will be submitted to EMA in London. There is no choice to submit only the MAA for several EU MSs.
For the coordination of the procedure the EMA adopts one CHMP member as Rapporteur as well as a second CHMP member as Co-Rapporteur. The applicant can make proposals for the choice of the Rapporteur and Co-Rapporteur, but finally the CHMP will decide who will be Rapporteur and Co-Rapporteur.
In comparison to MRP and DCP only one MAH is used within the CP (MAH identical in all MSs). This MAH is also only mentioned on the folding box of the medicinal product within the EU.
In addition the complete labeling (SPC, PIL, packaging materials) are content wise identical but have to be translated in all 23 national languages (including Norway and Iceland). National requirements (like national contact point, package size) can be mentioned simply in the so-called "blue- box".
Co-promotion is not possible for CP authorized product but as mentioned before in the "blue-box" the national contact person can be mentioned.
If co-marketing is intended a new registration is necessary. As Co-marketing partner for a CP authorized product a partner is needed who is represented in all 25 EU MSs. This can be seen as discrimination of middle-sized businesses as they often are not represented in all 25 MSs.
The basis fee for a CP application for which a full dossier needs to be presented are 254100 € (25500 € fee for each additional strength or pharmaceutical form including one presentation, submitted at the same time as the initial application for authorization, 6400 € for each additional presentation of the same strength and pharmaceutical form, submitted at the same time as the initial application for authorization). In case a CP application for which a full dossier needs not be presented the fees is only 164200 €. The registration costs for the CP are therefore higher compared to MRP and DCP.

Another issue at the CP is the danger with the trade name. For a CP it is mandatory that the applicant has a trademark which is accepted in all 25 EU MSs. For this it is absolutely advisable to make a "trademark-check" at the EMA (according to drug law). In addition it is mandatory that the applicant may ask for protection of the trademark at the European trademark office in Alicante.

Until Q4, 2005 (the date of submission is crucial for the application of the data protection periods) the data protection of the dossier are generally 10 years from first MA onwards for all products authorized through CP or ex-concertation procedure. At the MRP/DCP the data protection varies between 6 and 10 years depending on the EU MSs (10 years for national MAs granted by the following EU MSs: Belgium, Germany, France, Italy, the Netherlands, Sweden, UK and Luxemburg; 6 years for national MAs granted by the following EU MSs: Austria, Denmark, Finland, Ireland, Portugal, Spain, Greece, Poland, Czech Republic, Hungary, Lithuania, Latvia, Slovenia, Slovakia, Malta, Estonia, Cyprus and also Norway, Liechtenstein and Iceland).

The new protection periods of '8+2+1' are applicable only for reference medicinal products for which the MAA has been submitted as of 30 October 2005 for MRP, DCP and national procedures and as of 20 November 2005 for CP according to the revised Community Legislation. Directive 2004/27/EC[4], amending Directive 2001/83/EC[3], and Regulation (EC) No 726/2004[2] have introduced new rules concerning the periods, from the initial MA of the reference product, during which generic product applicants cannot rely on the dossier of the reference product for the purposes of submitting an application, obtaining MA or placing the product on the market.

Generic companies are allowed to submit their MAAs (which leads to the granting of a MA) after 8 years - this period is called "data exclusivity" but the launch of the product is first allowed after 10 years – this period of 10 years is called "market exclusivity". These periods are applicable for national procedures, MRP, DCP and CP authorized products.

The applicant has the possibility to extend the market exclusivity period for 1 additional year ('8+2+1') if within the first 8 years an indication enlargement or a new indication is granted via CP, MRP or DCP. It is essential that the MA of the new therapeutic indication within the first 8 years represents a significant clinical benefit in comparison with the existing therapies. The additional year of market protection is applicable for the global MA for the reference medicinal product. Generic products, with or without the new therapeutic indication, may not be placed on the market until expiry of the eleventh year.

The big advantage for the CP is that at the end of the evaluation phase one scientific opinion from the all EU MSs and finally one commission decision which is valid for EU, Norway, Iceland and Liechtenstein is received.

In case a negative CHMP opinion and as consequence a negative commission decision is made the applicant has the possibility to ask for an appeal procedure. During the appeal a new Rapporteur and Co-Rapporteur out of the CHMP members are appointed. The newly selected Rapporteur and Co-Rapporteur evaluate the same dossier as in the original procedure again. It is not allowed to submit new data during the appeal procedure. At the end of the appeal procedure a CHMP opinion and a commission decision is issued. This is then the final decision. There is not the possibility to make an appeal again.

In case in the CP a negative decision is made this is associated with a prohibition to market the medicinal product in the complete EU.

Another possibility is the opportunity to withdraw the MAA as soon as a negative decision threat. The applicant has then the possibility to submit a new MAA after updating the dossier via CP or maybe (depending on the product) via MRP or DCP.

In the MRP and DCP the applicant can choose the EU MSs where he will apply for a registration.

Another difference between the CP and DCP and MRP is the decision about the prescribing status ("prescription only") of a medicinal product. During the CP it is decided whether a medicinal product is prescription only or not. In comparison, during the MRP and DCP the prescription status is not decided as this decision is made by each MS nationally. This means that a harmonization of the prescribing status of a medicinal product during an MRP or DCP is nearly impossible. In addition there is only in Germany the § 49 German Drug Law ("Arzneimittelgesetz") (AMG) with an automatically obligation for medicinal product as prescribing drugs.

MRP or DCP:

The MRP can be used for MAAs of new as well as well-known substances. In general the applicant applies for an MAA in one particular MS - the so-called RMS. The national MAA in the RMS should take 210 days. After the granting of the MA in the RMS, the MRP can be started. The applicant will submit the MAA dossier to the selected CMSs (the applicant can choose the CMSs, there is no obligation to file the MA in all EU MSs). As basis for the mutual recognition of the CMSs the AR of the RMS is used. The RMS acts as mediator during the MRP.

The DCP offers an alternative to the MRP and applies where a medicinal product has not previously been granted a MA at the time of application. The main procedural difference between the MRP and DCP is that for a DCP an initial MA is not issued by the RMS. Instead of this, the CMSs participate early in the registration process by contributing to the preparation of the AR by the RMS. This AR builds the basis for the RMS and CMSs (the applicant can choose the CMSs, there is no obligation to go to all EU MSs) to agree the terms for authorization. Compared to the MRP also the timelines are different. The applicant submits the MAA to the RMS. By day 70 the RMS forwards the preliminary AR, SPC, PIL and labeling to the CMSs and to the applicant. Then the RMS and CMSs have time until day 105 to reach a consensus by updating the preliminary AR to become final AR, SPC, PL and labeling. Then the procedure is closed. In case no consensus between RMS and CMSs is reached at day 105 it might be possible to get a consensus until day 120 after resolution of minor points by updating the preliminary AR to become final AR, SPC, PIL and labeling.

If no consensus is possible at all the RMS will stop the clock at day 105 and ask the applicant to answer the open questions within three months. After valid submission of the answers to the questions from RMS and CMSs the RMS will start the clock at day 106 again. Then the RMS will update the preliminary AR to prepare a draft AR, draft SPC, draft PIL and labeling and will forward the documents to CMS. If by day 120 consensus is reached the procedure will be closed. After the closure of the procedure the CMSs have 30 day period to grant the MA (subject to acceptable translations).

One advantage of the MRP or DCP is that the applicant can choose the RMS. Also the CMSs can be chosen and there is no obligation to register the product in all 25 EU MSs. Therefore the procedure is often less complex regarding the numbers of translations as market potential is often seen only in a few MSs and only in these MSs submissions are then made. Based on this also the costs for the procedure are cheaper compared to CP.

The MRP or DCP can be repeated until all 25 EU MS are included. There is also the possibility to withdraw certain MSs from the MRP or DCP without withdrawal of the whole procedure. Within a MRP or DCP at maximum 25 national registrations in 25 EU MSs are possible. The SPC is identical in all EU MSs whereas the PIL is not harmonized (i.e. PIL can differ from MS to MS due to national requirements). Also as mentioned before the prescription status is not regulated through the MRP.

In addition at a MRP or DCP different MAHs are possible (from 1 to 25 different MAHs). Also co-promotion and co-marketing are possible without any issue for MRP or DCP products. In addition there is the possibility to transfer MAs e.g. to license holders.

For products authorized via MRP or DCP also different trademarks are possible. Through the usage of different trademarks within the different countries in the EU a better protection against parallel- and re-import is given.

A disadvantage for the MRP or DCP in the past (until Q4, 2005) was the fact that the data protection in the different EU/EEA states are between 6 and 10 years. The time of data protection starts with the first grant of a MA in the EU. In some EU MSs the data protection takes only 6 years (e.g. Denmark) whereas in other EU MSs (e.g. Germany) the data projection takes 10 years. Therefore this is very heterogeneous and not harmonized. Meanwhile this disadvantage is compensated as the general protection period '8+2+1' is homogenous for MRP, DCP and CP since October 2005.

In case the applicant has to choose between CP and MRP/DCP I would recommend using the MRP/DCP.

The MRP or DCP offers the applicant more flexibility and more options (please refer to advantages and disadvantages mentioned above).

The applicant has the opportunity to choose the RMS. It is recommended to choose a RMS which have a good and profound scientific standing for the specific indication in the EU and can defend the product during the MRP or DCP. Another important aspect for the choice of a RMS is the fact how fast the registration times for the MRP or DCP is to be able to start the MRP or go on with DCP as fast as possible. Another factor might be the fact to choose the country as RMS which needs the medicinal product mostly or choose the country which might have the biggest market potential (biggest business volume). The advantage of the MRP is the fact that the applicant can market the product already in the RMS after the approval even the MRP is still ongoing. The import to other countries is also possible.

The accelerated procedures are mostly only possible for medicinal products for life-threatening diseases which address unmet medical needs.

Croatia:
In Croatia it depends on the type of product which procedure can be used. As Croatia is member of nCADREAC and has adopted and implemented the EU legislation the same prerequisites for the different registration procedures applies as in EU. The applicant has to use the same procedure for applying a MA as it was done in EU. It means if a product is authorized via CP in EU, the nCADREAC procedure for products authorized in EU via CP has to be used in Croatia and if a product is authorized via MRP or DCP in EU, the nCADREAC procedure for products authorized in EU via MRP or DCP has to be used. The identical dossiers as submitted in EU including all answers

to questions, ARs and final approval letters or commission decision has to be submitted in Croatia. Therefore the applicant has no real choice for the procedure as it is binding due to the used EU procedure. Sometimes applicants might be concerned about confidentiality of the dossiers while submitting them in Croatia but in fact as the identical dossier is requested and a statement to confirm this has to be submitted there is no real alternative if the applicant would like to get a registration in Croatia.

China:

In China there are two registration procedures - the normal registration procedure and in addition the accelerated procedure called special review procedure. This special review procedure is only possible as long as no MA for this medicinal product is granted worldwide and only possible for new medicinal products (NCEs or NBEs) which are used for treatment of AIDS, malignant tumor and/or rare disease and which have obvious clinical therapeutically advantages and for new medicinal products which treat diseases for which there is no effective therapy. The advantage of special review procedure will be lost once the drug is approved in any country worldwide and it might be in reality quite unrealistic that China might be the first country who issues the MA for a new product especially as the registration time is quite long and special clinical date are needed (e.g. like local studies). The advantage in case of review times for the accelerated procedure is only 1.5 months compared to standard procedure. Another advantage of this special review procedure is the fact that rolling submission is allowed (e.g. safety, stability, CMC development, etc.). The biggest advantage of this special review procedure is the fact that pre- and in-process consultation at CDE during the NDA review process is permitted, so the applicant has to the opportunity to be in close contact with CDE during the review process. This is not possible for the standard review procedure. Based on the differences between special and standard review procedure the applicant has to evaluate for a new product very carefully whether a special review procedure is possible - whether all prerequisites are fulfilled. In case all prerequisites for applying of special review procedure are fulfilled the applicant has to decide whether to use this procedure. It might be useful to do the first submission of MAA in China in order to use the special review procedure. In this case a very good planning regarding submission of MAs in different countries has to be made to ensure that China is the first country who issues the MA.

Conclusion of different registration procedures in the different countries:

In most of the countries different registration procedures exist. The different registration procedures have often well defined prerequisites under which circumstances which type of registration procedure can be used (please refer to the table "Comparison of different registration procedures in the different countries and pro/con arguments for each procedure" page 95 ff) - so it is mostly not possible for the applicant to choose by themselves the type of registration procedure. The accelerated procedures are in some countries only possible for MAAs of NCEs and not for NBEs due to the complexity of NBEs. In most countries fast track procedures are only applicable for serious or life-threatening disease which have potential to address unmet medical need or for life-saving drugs or only for orphan drugs. The "normal" registration procedures are applicable for all kind of products and can be used by the applicant for all kind of MAAs. Therefore it is advisable that the applicant evaluates very carefully before submission of an MAA which type of registration procedure can be used in which country for which type of product. In case of doubt or open questions it is advisable that the applicant may ask for a consultation meeting with the authority of the concerned country. After the registration procedures are chosen for each country the applicant can submit the MAA.

5 Development of the Global Regulatory Strategy for a New Marketing Authorization Application for a New Compound

In the following chapter the development of a new compound (NBE or NCE) will be described and the main differences between the development of an NBE and an NCE will be addressed shortly. In addition a regulatory strategy for an NBE on the example of a mAb is provided. The development of a new compound (NBE or NCE) in general as well as for the proposed regulatory strategy for an NBE described here on the example of a mAb is based on my personal experience in pharmaceutical industry.

5.1 Development of a New Compound

This chapter is based on own experience and research in pharmaceutical industry for several years.
The global development of a new compound (NBE or NCE) is divided in several stages:

- CMC development
- Nonclinical development
- Clinical development

The whole development for a global compound which should be submitted and approved worldwide should be based on the existing ICH guidelines for quality (quality (Q) guidelines), nonclinical (safety (S) guidelines) and clinical (efficacy (E) guidelines) and if applicable the multidisciplinary (M) guidelines. In addition to the applicable ICH guidelines it is important to take also some national guidelines into consideration e.g. stability guidelines (especially guidelines for stability data for climatic zone III, IVA and IVB) or some clinical guidelines.
At the beginning of a global development of a new compound it is advisable to create a global plan covering a short summary for the development of a new compound with regard to quality, nonclinical and clinical (divided into the different indications in development). Additionally trademark issues, IP issues and regulatory issues need to be mentioned within the global plan. In addition product objectives (short term, midterm and long term objectives) and marketing aspects (e.g. financial analysis like sales forecast for the indications in development) and financial aspects (like costs for research and development, cost of goods or net present value) should be mentioned within this global plan. This global plan contains also the key risks as well as

opportunities for the development. It is recommended to make a so called SWOT analysis (Strengths, Weakness, Opportunities and Threats) for the whole development. In addition it is recommended to provide for each section within this global plan a short risk analysis (risks and opportunities). This global plan will not contain all mentioned sections at the beginning of development but will grow during the development and will be updated with new aspects and information. In parallel or shortly after the creation of the global plan the global route map should be created (e.g. as excel or MS project file). This global route map should cover the main goals for all areas (like quality, nonclinical, clinical) of the development from starting of development until approval of MAA and launch of the product with the approx. timelines for the different phases and tasks of the development.

In addition to this global plan and the global route map it is recommended to prepare development plans for the different areas of development, i.e. one quality development plan, one nonclinical development plan and one clinical development plan. The timing for the creation of the quality development plan, nonclinical development plan and clinical development plan differs based on status of development. First the quality and nonclinical development plans will be created as these areas are first in the development of a new compound. It is important that at least the main part of the nonclinical development should be finalized before the clinical development is started. Before starting the clinical development the clinical development plan will be created. Based on the clinical development plan also a regulatory development plan with the submission strategy should be created. The regulatory development plan contains the main regulatory strategy, the relevant regulations and guidelines to be considered, risk analysis and recommendations. It is also advisable to include some information on competitive products if available. Within the regulatory development plan shortly the CMC strategy, nonclinical strategy as well as the clinical strategy is summarized to build based on them the regulatory strategy.

In parallel or shortly after the creation of the different development plans, route maps for each of different development areas (one route map for quality, one for nonclinical, one for clinical and one for regulatory) with the main goals, tasks and timelines (e.g. excel or MS project can be used) will be created.

The global plan, the global route map as well as the development plans for the different areas of development and the route maps for the different development areas are living documents and need to be updated during the different development phases. To be able to create such a global plan and to ensure the proper development of a new compound a global development team should be created. This global development team should consist at least of representatives from the following functions: one representative from CMC, one representative from nonclinical (ideally one from toxicology and one from pharmacology), one representative from clinical, one representative from regulatory affairs and one representative from marketing. In addition the team should be led by a team leader and should have also one project manager as member for all project coordinating work. The adequate time point for creation of such a global development team is after finalization of Phase 0 - before starting with clinical trials. This team might be later in development get some additional team member based on the necessity, e.g. somebody from drug safety, biomarker department, commercial department, pricing department, legal department or trademark department. This global development team will prepare the global plan and the global route map with the support of the different involved functions.

Based on the global development team it is recommended to build up some "subteams" in order to ensure a good communication line and easy decision making processes. These subteams should be divided by the functions, e.g. one CMC subteam, one nonclinical subteam, one clinical subteam and one regulatory subteam. These subteams should also prepare their plans (i.e. CMC development plan, nonclinical development plan, clinical development plan and regulatory development plan). It is advisable that within these subteams also the global team leader or at least the project manager of the global team is a permanent member in order to ensure the consistency of the project and for coordination of the project. One of the subteams is the CMC subteam led by the CMC representative of the global team. The CMC subteam should consist of the different functions of CMC (e.g. pharmaceutical development unit, analytical /QC unit, clinical trial supply unit, quality assurance unit, qualified person) as well as one representative of regulatory affairs and the global team leader or at least one project manager of the global team. The major points which are discussed in such a subteam can then be transferred via the leader of the subteam to the global team.

There should be a nonclinical subteam led by the nonclinical representative of the global team. The nonclinical subteam should consist of the different functions of nonclinical (e.g. toxicology, pharmacokinetic, pharmacodynamics, biomarkers) as well as one representative of regulatory affairs and the global team leader or at least one project manager of the global team.

In addition there should be established a clinical subteam led by the clinical representative of the global team. The clinical subteam should consist of the different areas of clinical (e.g. clinical operations, drug safety, maybe different clinicians (based on different indications), data management, statistics) as well as one representative of regulatory affairs and the global team leader or at least one project manager of the global team.

In addition there should also be established a regulatory subteam led by the regulatory representative of the global team. The regulatory subteam should consist of the different functions of regulatory (e.g. regulatory therapeutical area (who is normally the representative in the global team), regulatory operations, labeling, and regulatory international).

The most important points which are discussed in such a subteam can then be transferred via the leader of the subteams to the global team for information and also for decision making.

Additional subteams might be established based on the status of development and the necessity seen by the global team. It is important to have these teams and subteams in order to ensure an easy communication flow (that everybody who needs to be informed is informed) and that also the decision making process can be handled quite easily. In general the global team has to make the final decisions for the project. Sometimes, especially for the critical strategic and cost intensive decisions (like "go" for Phase III study or not), it is necessary that the global team has to ask the upper management for final confirmation and agreement of their decisions/proposals.

In general the described steps, plans and activities needed are valid for the development of NCE as well as an NBE. The main differences between the development of an NCE and an NBE appear in the CMC development as the CMC development for an NCE is different from an NBE (please refer to CMC development plan).

In the following the different recommended development plans will be discussed in more details:

CMC development plan:
All aspects regarding the CMC development should be covered. The plan should be prepared and updated by the CMC subteam.

The whole CMC development will be done according to ICH guidelines and requirements ("Q" ICH guidelines) in order to be able to receive MAs in ICH region as well as in many non-ICH-countries as a lot of non-ICH countries following ICH requirements. In addition some national regulations and guidelines may be taken into consideration (e.g. stability requirements for ASEAN countries or stability requirements for some LA countries regarding climatic zones III and IVA/IVB) in order to capture all needed requirements to be able to get MAs in all countries worldwide.

Within the CMC development plan the CMC development strategy is described which includes the objective of the CMC development program as well as the development strategy.

It is important to have the final formulation which is intended for submission of MAA ready before starting the Phase III trials.

All guidelines and regulations with regard to stability requirements should be taken into consideration in order to be able to roll-out the MAA with all requested data to all countries worldwide.

At the end of the plan there should be a decision tree to be able to decide for go/no go based on results of the proposed study program and short explanation for go/no go criteria should be provided.

This decision tree contains also so called "Decision points". One of these points is the decision to start the nonclinical development based on the results and the compound identified so far. If the results are promising the decision will be positive and the nonclinical development will be started. Based on experiences normally at the beginning of CMC development there are 100 compounds from which maybe 15-20 compounds (15-20%) will pass this first decision point and will go into nonclinical development.

At the beginning of a development of a new compound there are a lot of laboratory actions needed to find first a compound which can be further development. If this compound is found then the preclinical development will be started. In this stage normally not the final formulation of the DP is available but a so-called "pre" formulation. During the preclinical development also the CMC development is ongoing to develop other formulations, e.g. more stable or better compliant formulations for animals and humans. The final formulation should be available before starting the Phase III clinical studies in order to perform the pivotal Phase III studies with the final formulation which will be then also submitted to apply for the MA. In certain cases it is sometimes needed to also make changes at the formulation during Phase III clinical studies. These changes should be discussed with the authorities before submitting the changes in an IND amendment (USA) or CTA amendment (EU) to the authority.

In general the described steps, plans and activities needed are valid for the development of NCE as well as an NBE. The main differences between the development of an NCE and an NBE appear in the CMC development as the CMC development for an NCE is different from an NBE. An NCE is a clear defined molecule whereas an NBE consists of a more complex structure. The influence of the manufacturing process on the molecule/substance needs also to be considered. An NCE is defined by the product itself whereas an NBE is not only defined by the product itself but also by the manufacturing process. Therefore the manufacturing processes of an NCE and an NBE differ. Each single change at the manufacturing process of an NBE might have therefore a big impact on the molecule whereas changes at the manufacturing process for an NCE will have no or only very little influence on the product.

One critical topic regarding the CMC development of an NCE is often the definition of the starting material for the manufacturing process. Another critical issue especially for NCEs are the impurities. The impurities have to be characterized and analyzes very detailed according to the valid guidelines. It is strongly recommended to discuss such topics in advance with the authorities.

Nonclinical development plan:
All aspects regarding the nonclinical development should be covered. The plan should be prepared and updated by the nonclinical subteam.

The whole nonclinical development will be done according to ICH guidelines and requirements ("S" ICH guidelines) in order to get MAs in ICH region as well as in many non-ICH-countries as a lot of non-ICH countries follow ICH requirements. In addition some national regulations and guidelines may be taken into consideration in order to capture all needed requirements to be able to get MAs in all countries worldwide.

Within the nonclinical development plan the nonclinical development strategy is described which includes the objective of the nonclinical development program as well as the development strategy.

All requested toxicological studies should be performed before starting the clinical development.

If combination products are under development combination toxicological studies should be taken into consideration (especially if the single compounds are quite toxic). If no experience with the combination of products exists it is advisable to perform a combination toxicological study. In case of some doubts it might be helpful to ask for an authority meeting to clarify this question.

At the end of the nonclinical development plan there should be a decision tree to be able to decide for go/no go based on results of the proposed study program and short explanation for go/no go criteria should be provided.

This decision tree contains also so called "Decision points". One of these points is for sure the decision to go on with clinical development based on the results of the nonclinical studies. If the results are promising the decision will be positive and the clinical development will be started.

Based on experiences normally at the beginning of CMC development there are 100 compounds from which maybe 15-20 compounds (15-20%) will pass this first decision point and will go into nonclinical development. Based on the results of the nonclinical development maybe 2-3 compounds (max. 10-15% out of nonclinical development) will then pass the second decision point and go into the clinical development.

Clinical development plan:

All aspects regarding the clinical development should be covered. The plan should be prepared and updated by the clinical subteam.

The whole clinical development will be done according to ICH guidelines and requirements ("E" ICH guidelines) in order to receive MAs in ICH region as well as in many non-ICH-countries as a lot of non-ICH countries following ICH requirements. In addition some national regulations and guidelines (e.g. Chinese regulation or regulation from Brazil or Turkey) might be taken into consideration in order to capture all needed requirements to be able to get MAs in all countries worldwide.

Within the clinical development plan the clinical development strategy is described which includes the objective of the clinical development program as well as the development strategy. The main part of the clinical development part is covered with the detailed clinical considerations divided into:

- Choice of endpoints
- Choice of design and objectives
- Choice of population
- Choice of dose and dosing regimen
- Choice of control group
- Number of subjects and duration of exposure
- Trial design issues
- Statistical issues
- Safety issues
- Regulatory issues
- Pediatric investigational plan (PIP)
- Other issues

Besides the clinical consideration also information for the health economics strategy as well as medical affairs strategy should be included into the plan. Some considerations regarding biomarkers which become more and more important in order to be able to develop patient tailored medicinal drugs should be included into the clinical development plan. At the end of the plan there should be a decision tree to be able to decide for go/no go based on results of the proposed study program and short explanation for go/no go criteria should be provided.

This decision tree contains also so called "Decision points". Within the clinical development plan there should be two very important decision points. The first decision point should be after finalization of Phase II studies. If the results of the performed Phase I and Phase II studies are promising and positive the clinical development should go on and the pivotal Phase III studies should be initiated. In case the results are only borderline or even negative it should be very carefully evaluated whether clinical development should go on or should be stopped.

The second important decision point with the clinical development is after finalization of Phase III trials. Based on the results of the pivotal Phase III studies it should be decided whether to apply for a MA or not. In case the results of the performed Phase III studies are positive and meet their endpoints the dossier should be prepared to be able to apply for a MA. In case the results are only borderline or even negative it should be very carefully evaluated whether a MA submission should be done and whether the development should go on or should be stopped.

Based on a lot of experiences normally at the beginning of CMC development there are 100 compounds from which maybe 15-20 compounds (15-20%) will pass the first decision point and will go into nonclinical development. Based on the results of the nonclinical development maybe 2-3 compounds (max. 10-15% out of nonclinical development) will then pass the second decision point and go on into the clinical development. The third decision point within the clinical development whether to initiate Phase III studies based on results of Phase I and II studies normally pass only maximum one compound. This means in total that normally only 1 % of the compounds which started in the CMC development will pass all decision points and will go in Phase III clinical trials and have the chance to get a MA and can be launched and marketed after successful registration.

Regulatory development plan:

All aspects regarding the regulatory development should be covered. The plan should be prepared and updated by the regulatory subteam.

The regulatory development plan is mostly based on the clinical development plan. Therefore it is recommended to establish first the clinical development plan and afterwards the regulatory development plan.

Within the regulatory development plan a summary of the project is provided as well as the regulatory issues, risk assessment and recommendations. All available and to be considered guidelines and regulations are mentioned, divided into quality guidelines, nonclinical and clinical guidelines. It is recommended to include also some regulatory information on competitive products as well as information on combination partners for the new compound if applicable. Also some information regarding the cooperation with license partners, if applicable should be included in the regulatory development plan. Shortly there should the supply chain strategy as well as the nonclinical and clinical development strategy be mentioned based on the CMC, nonclinical and clinical development plans.

Then the regulatory development plan should have a chapter with all the regulatory activities like clinical trial licenses, import licenses, manufacturing licenses, orphan drug applications (if applicable), fast track status (if applicable), authority advice strategy (like scientific advices), DMFs and CEPs, master data sheet preparation, application for INN/ United States Adopted Name (USAN), Anatomical Therapeutic Chemical / Defined Daily Dose Classification (ATC code), pediatric trials and roll-out strategy to countries worldwide. The MA strategy chapter contains target indications, timing of submissions in the different regions, dossier type, electronic submissions, project plan creation, application fees and the regional strategies for initial MAA (in EU, USA, SEA,...). Finally a short chapter regarding life cycle management should be included (which might be created and filled with content first during the development phases).

If the regulatory strategy and the corresponding timelines for the MA submission are fixed in the regulatory development plan, the next steps can be initiated. Based on the planned submission timelines a submission team should be created latest 1 year (better 1,5 or 2 years) before planned first submission of the MAA. This team consists of representatives of the different disciplines (from CMC, nonclinical, clinical and regulatory) who are responsible for creating the MA dossier for submission of the MAA to the authorities. The representatives of the different disciplines are the authors of the different CTD sections of the dossier. Besides the authors of the documents for the MA dossier also a representative from marketing, pricing and the global team leader or one of the project managers of the global team should be members of the submission team in order to follow and to implement the submission strategy accordingly. The submission team will create a route map containing all CTD documents, authors and timelines for preparing the different sections of a dossier (example of such a route map, see APPENDIX 17).

As EU and USA are still the most important markets the submission normally will be made first in these two countries. Therefore the submission team works first for the submissions in EU and USA. But as also other countries gets more and more important also the preparations for the other countries should be started. Therefore a submission strategy for the roll-out to the other countries is initiated ideally already in the regulatory development plan or even during the preparation of dossier for the first MA submissions in EU and USA.

In the following the regulatory strategy for an NBE on the example of a mAb is presented. To be able to develop a regulatory strategy and a submission strategy first a short description of a mAb is provided to be able to develop for this kind of medicinal product a global regulatory strategy.

It is important to know that there is not only one definition of a biotech product. For the purpose of this dissertation a biotech product is a medicinal product manufactured by genetically modified micro-organisms or cell lines (refer to Ph. Eur. monograph on Products of recombinant DNA technology). Such products also fall under the definition of the EU Regulation 726/2004[2] and include drugs like mAbs.

The differences between the submission strategy for an NBE and an NCE are shortly discussed at the end of the summary and discussion section (please refer to 5.5. Summary and Discussion).

5.2 Short Introduction of a Monoclonal Antibody

First a short description of a mAb is provided to be able to develop for this kind of medicinal product a global regulatory strategy.

5.2.1 Definition

A mAb is a specific antibody which is made by one type of immune cell. These immune cells are all clones of a unique parent cell.

"Monoclonal antibodies (mAb or moAb) are monospecific antibodies that are the same because they are made by one type of immune cell which are all clones of a unique parent cell. Given almost any substance, it is possible to create monoclonal antibodies that specifically bind to that substance; they can then serve to detect or purify that

substance. This has become an important tool in biochemistry, molecular biology and medicine. When used as medications, the non-proprietary drug name ends in -mab."[57]

5.2.2 Antibody structure

Antibodies consist of four polypeptide chains held together by disulfide bonds:
The two heavy chains are made up of the VH domain and 3 constant regions.
The two light chains are made up of the VL domain and one constant region.
The constant regions have a conserved amino acid sequence and exhibit low variability. [57]

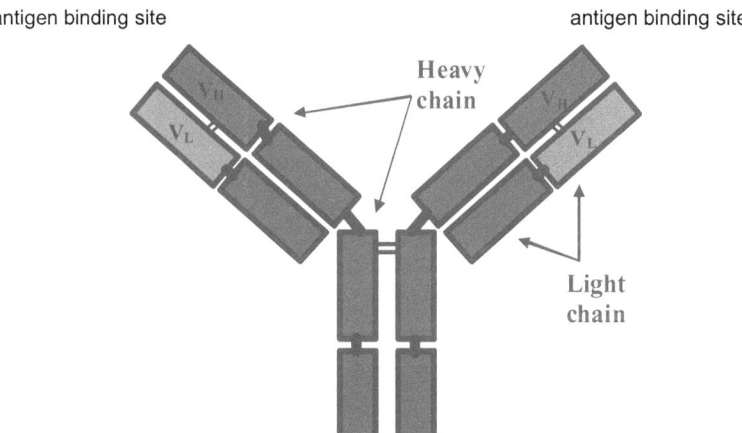

5.2.3 Antibody Function

Antibodies have two major functions: [57]

- Recognize and bind antigen
- Induce immune responses after binding

The variable region mediates binding

- Affinity for a given antigen is determined by the variable region
- The variable region confers absolute specificity for an antigen

The constant region mediates immune response after binding

- Different classes of constant regions generate different isotypes
- Different isotypes of antibody have differing properties

---

[57] http://en.wikipedia.org/wiki/Monoclonal_antibodies - dated 10.05.2010

5.2.4 Types of Monoclonal Antibodies

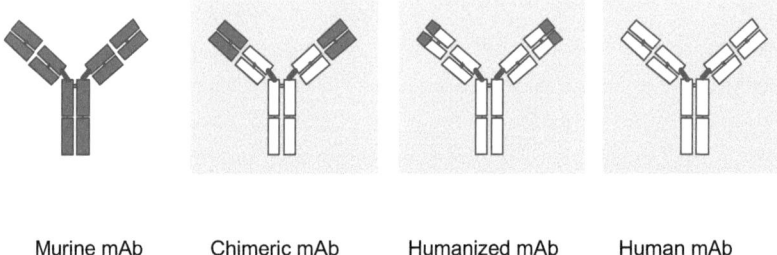

Murine mAb   Chimeric mAb   Humanized mAb   Human mAb

Murine mAb:

- Consists only of murine cells
- High incidence of hypersensitivity
- High levels of neutralizing antibodies

The murine mAbs are quite similar to the human mAbs but not completely identical. Therefore the human immune system recognizes mouse antibodies as foreign and rapidly removing them from circulation and causing systemic inflammatory effects. Such responses are recognized as producing HACA (human anti-chimeric antibodies) or HAMA (human anti-mouse antibodies). Therefore murine mAbs have a high incidence of hypersensitivity reactions. The solution would be to generate human antibodies directly from humans. This would mean that human have to be treated with antigens in order to produce antibodies. This is generally not seen as ethical therefore the companies tried to find other solutions to create "more" human like antibodies.

One possible approach is that DNA is taken that encodes the binding protein of monoclonal mouse antibodies and is merged with human antibody-producing DNA. Normally mammalian cell cultures are used to express this DNA and produce these half-mouse and half-human antibodies. Depending how big the part of the mouse antibody is used, it is a chimeric or a humanized antibody. [57]

Chimeric mAb:

- The variable region of the mAb consists of murine cells, the rest of the mAb consists of human cells
- Quite high incidence for hypersensitivity
- Low levels of neutralizing antibodies

Humanized mAb:

- Only the upper ends of the variable regions of the mAb consists of murine cells, the rest of the mAb consists of human cells
- Hypersensitivity is lower compared to murine or chimeric mAbs but still possible
- Low levels of neutralizing antibodies

In newer times scientists were successful to create "fully" human antibodies in order to avoid some of side effects of chimeric or humanized antibodies. Two successful approaches were identified: [57]

- phage display-generated antibodies
- mice genetically engineered to produce more human-like antibodies

Human mAb:

- The complete mAb consists of human cells
- Incidence for hypersensitivity is very low
- Low levels of neutralizing antibodies [57]

5.2.5 Goals of Monoclonal Antibodies

- Activity
    - High specificity for a target critical to tumor growth and survival
    - Able to achieve meaningful clinical benefit
- Utility
    - Can be used as single agent or in combination
    - Minimal overlapping toxicities
    - Potential targets present across tumor types and stages of disease

For cancer there are currently several treatment options:

	MAbs	Tyrosine Kinase Inhibitors	Chemo-therapy	Radiation
Specificity for target	Absolute specificity	Variable specificity	Low specificity	Low specificity
Toxicity	Low	Low/moderate	High	Moderate
Administration	IV	IV/oral	IV/oral	Local
Half-life	Days to weeks	Hours to days	Hours to days	NA

5.2.6 Cancer Treatment

As mentioned above one big field for mAbs is the option as cancer treatment. If used as cancer treatment mAbs *"bind only to cancer cell-specific antigens and induce an immunological response against the target cancer cell. Such mAb could also be modified for delivery of a toxin, radioisotope, cytokine or other active conjugate; it is also possible to design bispecific antibodies that can bind with their Fab regions both to target antigen and to a conjugate or effector cell. In fact, every intact antibody can bind to cell receptors or other proteins with its Fc region."*[67]

Example for mAbs for cancer:

"*ADEPT, antibody directed enzyme prodrug therapy; ADCC, antibody dependent cell-mediated cytotoxicity; CDC, complement dependent cytotoxicity; MAb, monoclonal antibody; scFv, single-chain Fv fragment.*"[67]

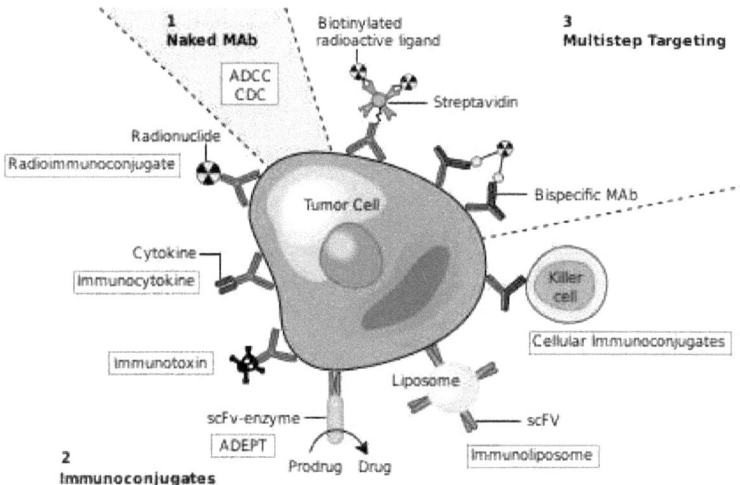

5.2.7 Conclusion Monoclonal Antibodies

- MAbs are excellent therapeutic agents in oncology
  - When used as a single agent or when used in combination
  - High specificity to target
  - Manageable side effect profile
- MAb engineering has evolved over time
  - Immune responses to murine antibodies led to the creation of chimeric, humanized, and human antibodies
  - Hypersensitivity has remained as a class effect of antibodies

5.2.8 Manufacturing Process of a New Biotech Product, Example of a Monoclonal Antibody

The next step after some general aspects of mAbs is to define a biotech product and to explain shortly the general manufacturing process of a mAb:

The main difference between an NCE and an NBE is the influence of the manufacturing process on the molecule/substance. An NCE is defined by the product itself whereas an NBE is not only defined by the product itself but also by the manufacturing process. Each single change at the manufacturing process of an NBE might have therefore a big impact on the molecule.

The general manufacturing process of an NBE as example of a mAb can be described as follows:

- First, an appropriate micro-organism or cell line has to be selected that is known to be able to manufacture similar proteins.

- These are usually either
  - Bacteria (e.g. E. coli) or
  - Yeast (e.g. Saccharomyces) or
  - Mammalian cell lines (e.g. Chinese Hamster Ovary [CHO] cells)

- Second, the gene sequence (vector) encoding for the desired protein needs to be inserted in the genome of the so-called host cell line

Transfection of cells[50]

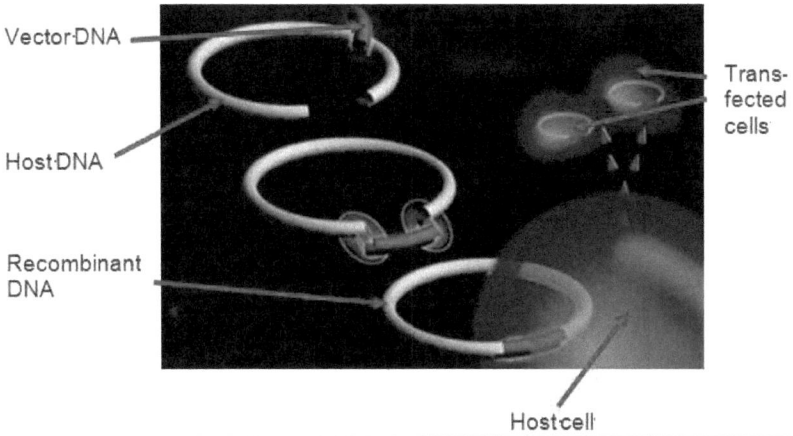

Vector DNA

Host DNA

Recombinant DNA

Trans-fected cells

Host cell

Glycosylation

- The genetic sequence defines the amino acid sequence of a protein
- However, many biotech drugs also contain complex carbohydrates, i.e. they are in essence glycoproteins not just proteins
- The process by which these carbohydrates are attached to the protein is called glycosylation
- Glycosylation often impacts on the biological activity, immunogenicity and pharmacokinetics of biotech drugs
- Glycosylation is usually very sensitive to manufacturing changes

Master Cell Bank (MCB)

- Once a cell line is identified which produces the desired protein in the required quality and quantity a so-called Master Cell Bank (MCB) is created, i.e.
- the cells are suspended in a defined storage medium (e.g. fetal calf serum) and equal amounts are distributed in vials (typically 200-300)
- These vials are then refrigerated in liquid nitrogen at -77 K (-196°C)
- MCB is usually stored at - 70°C or lower

- This MCB will be source of all material manufactured through the whole life-cycle of a drug, i.e. one MCB results in one product

To sum up there is a short general overview how to produce a mAb.

A general representation of the methods used to produce mAbs[58]

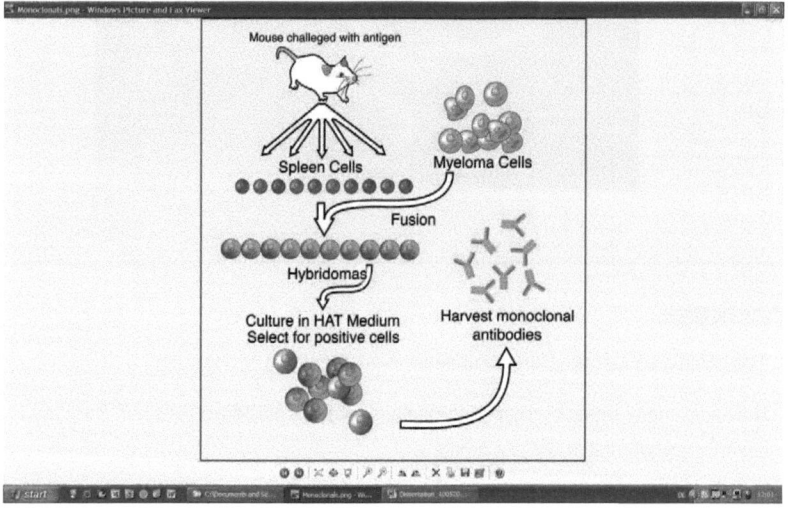

---

[58] http://en.wikipedia.org/wiki/Biomarker - dated 25.08.2010

General biotech manufacturing scheme[50]

Active pharmaceutical ingredient, Drug Substance

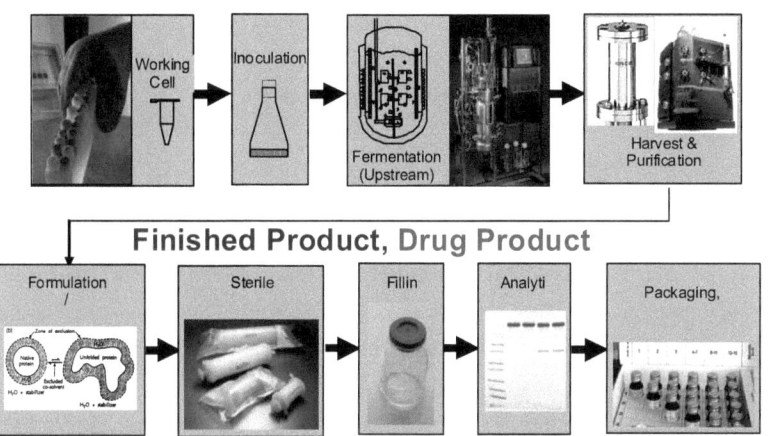

Finished Product, Drug Product

Conclusion:
A biotech product is defined not only by the product but also by the process. This is clearly reflected in the structure and content of the dossier for a biotech product.

5.3 Development of a Monoclonal Antibody

This chapter is based on my own experience in pharmaceutical industry for several years.
Based on the general development activities (see chapter 5.1) and the global plan (see APPENDIX 18) a regulatory strategy for a mAb called Monotuximab is developed. The development takes place in the indications squamous cell cancer of the head and neck (SCCHN), Hodgkin lymphoma and breast cancer.

5.3.1 Compound & Mode of Action

Monotuximab is a humanized mAb of the immunoglobulin G1 (IgG1) class targeting the human epidermal growth factor receptor (EGFR)." *The **epidermal growth factor receptor** (EGFR; ErbB-1; HER1 in humans) is the cell-surface receptor for members of the epidermal growth factor family (EGF-family) of extracellular protein ligands. The epidermal growth factor receptor is a member of the ErbB family of receptors, a subfamily of four closely related receptor tyrosine kinases: EGFR (ErbB-1), HER2/c-neu (ErbB-2), Her 3 (ErbB-3) and Her 4 (ErbB-4). Mutations affecting EGFR expression or activity could result in cancer.-EGFR exists on the cell surface and is activated by binding of its specific ligands, including epidermal growth factor and transforming growth factor α (TGFα).*[59]

Compared to chemotherapy Monotuximab specifically targets and binds to EGFR. This binding inhibits the activation of the receptor and the subsequent signal-transduction pathway. The results of this inhibition are a reduction of the invasion of normal tissues by tumor cells and the spread of tumors to new sites. It is also believed to inhibit the ability of tumor cells to repair the damage caused by chemotherapy and radiotherapy and to inhibit the formation of new blood vessels inside tumors, which appears to lead to an overall suppression of tumor growth.

5.3.2 Development Objectives

- Registration of Monotuximab first in EU and USA and afterwards roll-out to JP and to non-ICH-countries for the indication SCCHN

- Finalize the ongoing clinical studies in Hodgkin lymphoma and breast cancer with positive results (meeting the endpoints)

- Registration of new indication Hodgkin lymphoma in ICH and non-ICH-countries after positive studies

- Registration of new indication breast cancer in ICH and non-ICH-countries after positive studies

- Establish Monotuximab as important part of the gold standard treatment regimens in tumors where EGFR is expressed

---

[59] *http://en.wikipedia.org/wiki/Epidermal_growth_factor_receptor*

5.4 Development of the Global Regulatory Strategy for a Monoclonal Antibody

This chapter is based on my own experience in pharmaceutical industry for several years.

5.4.1 Executive Summary of the Regulatory Strategy

The global regulatory strategy for the mAb Monotuximab is focused on achieving fastest path to market in EU and US followed by other important markets. The initial filing is planned for the indication SCCHN, most commonly known as head and neck cancer. SCCHN represents 95% of all head & neck cancers and is associated with a very poor prognosis. SCCHN is characterized by a high EGFR expression rate of 90-100%. There is a high unmet medical need in the treatment of SCCHN comprising

- improved survival of patients with recurrent and/or metastatic disease
- enhancement of radiotherapy
- need for new treatment options
- higher response rates can minimize the surgery of early stage disease (organ preservation)

As mentioned above SCCHN represents an area of high unmet medical need and an orphan indication at least in USA, which allows access to favorable regulatory mechanisms, including fast track status and priority review as well as Orphan Drug Designation. In EU the indication SCCHN does not fall under the Orphan Drug Designation and also not under the accelerated registration procedure, so only the normal assessment procedure is possible in the EU.

Positive outcomes of the ongoing Phase II studies 001 and 002 will trigger the decision for a pivotal Phase III trial in SCCHN. The design of the pivotal Phase III trial will be discussed with FDA and EMA/CHMP, preferably via a parallel (harmonized) scientific advice.

The design of the pivotal Phase III trial in SCCHN might be complicated by potentially different opinions of EMA/CHMP and FDA with respect to clinical endpoint and comparator arm. FDA will most likely prefer a primary survival endpoint in SCCHN, whereas EMA/CHMP might consider a surrogate endpoint like progression-free survival (PFS) as a basis for approval. A potential pivotal trial in SCCHN is planned to be powered for a survival endpoint, which might offer the option for earlier approval based on a planned interim analysis with a surrogate endpoint like PFS. Thereby a single global study could potentially satisfy both EMA and FDA.

All guidelines which should be taken into consideration for the development are listed in APPENDIX 19.

As EU and USA are still the most important markets the submission will be made first in these two countries. Therefore the submission team works first for the submissions in EU and USA. But as also other countries gets more and more important also the preparations for the other countries should be started. Therefore a submission strategy for the roll-out to the other countries is initiated ideally already in the regulatory development plan or even during the preparation of dossier for the first MA submissions in EU and USA.

In the following the proposed submission strategy for roll-out to international (non-ICH) countries) for the developed mAb Monotuximab is presented:

5.4.2 Regulatory Activities
5.4.2.1 Clinical Trial Licenses

A Phase II study for the combination of Monotuximab and radiation in SCCHN is currently ongoing. Participating countries are Germany, Spain, France, Belgium, Portugal, UK, USA, CH, Russia, China, Taiwan, South Korea, Singapore, Brazil, Argentina, Venezuela, Chile and Mexico.

5.4.2.2 Orphan Drug Application

Monotuximab has been designated as an orphan medicinal product for the treatment of SCCHN in the USA in September 2006. Orphan product designation provides 7 years of marketing exclusivity in the US, and possible tax credits for development costs. In addition a waiver can be requested regarding the user fees for a MA in the US.

5.4.2.3 Fast Track Status

The application for fast track status in the US in SCCHN was granted in Q1, 2007. Fast track designation provides as described before more visibility and a higher level of commitment of FDA resources. It allows for greater access to FDA consultations and for a 'rolling submission' of portions of the MA as they become available which facilitates the FDA review process. The priority review process and accelerated approval strategies are available in addition to the fast track program.

5.4.2.4 Authority Advice Strategy

Positive outcomes of study 001 and 002 will trigger the decision for a pivotal Phase III trial in SCCHN. Open issues will then be discussed with the FDA at an End-of-Phase II meeting. CMC and clinical topics will most likely be addressed in separate meetings.

In addition there is the need for getting a feedback from EMA/CHMP, especially with respect to the design of a global pivotal clinical trial in SCCHN. Due to the possibility of different views of EMA/CHMP and FDA on endpoints and comparator the option for a parallel clinical scientific advice should be explored. The same information (study synopsis, etc.) will be submitted to both authorities including a cover letter allowing exchange of information between both parties. The context would be a request for an End-of-Phase II meeting with the FDA and for scientific advice with the EMA, respectively. CMC and non-clinical issues could also be covered by the EMA advice as appropriate, maybe as alternative also a separate meeting should be planned (as planned for USA). The timing of a parallel scientific advice will be critical since the EMA Scientific Advice Working Group meeting is only once a month. The FDA should therefore be informed at least 4 months before an anticipated joint meeting of the authorities. Following the harmonization of advice, the pivotal study protocol may be submitted to FDA for the Special Protocol Assessment (SPA) procedure, to provide a binding agreement for the pivotal trial and registration strategy.

Besides the meetings with EMA and USA also meetings with some national EU authorities should also be taken into consideration. These meetings with national EU authorities should not overlap from a timing point of view with a concurrent EMA advice procedure on the same topic. Consequently, once data from studies 001 and 002 become available, questions on the pivotal Phase III study design should only be discussed with national EU authorities before approaching the EMA. These meetings should be held with national EU authorities prior to taking a decision for the proposal of Rapporteur and Co-Rapporteur.

5.4.2.5 Marketing Authorization Strategy

Depending on the results of studies 001 and 002, a pivotal Phase III study is planned to achieve first registration in SCCHN in EU (via CP) and US.

5.4.2.6 Target Indications and Key Labeling Statements

Treatment of patients with SCCHN in combination with radiation therapy for locally advanced disease.

Monotuximab is used concomitantly with radiation therapy. It is recommended to start Monotuximab therapy one week before radiation therapy and to continue Monotuximab therapy until the end of the radiation therapy period.

Prior to the first infusion, patients must receive premedication with an antihistamine and a

corticosteroid. This premedication is recommended prior to all subsequent infusions.

Monotuximab is administered once every two weeks. The initial dose is 500 mg Monotuximab per m² body surface area. All subsequent weekly doses are 390 mg Monotuximab per m² each.

5.4.2.7 Timing of Submission in Regions

The marketing authorization strategy is focused on initial approval in SCCHN in EU and US. Parallel submissions in both regions are currently targeted for Q1,11. The approved indications will then be expanded to JP and non-ICH countries. For some countries also parallel submissions to EU and US are possible and will be evaluated whether to do or not.

5.4.2.8 Dossier Type

The initial applications in EU and US will be based on a dossier in CTD format.

5.4.2.9 Electronic Submission

The initial application in EU and US in 2011 is expected to be based on an eCTD submission.

5.4.3 Regional Strategies for Initial Application in ICH

As EU and USA are still the most important markets the preparation of the dossier will be first done for these two countries.

5.4.3.1 EU

The potential pivotal clinical trial in SCCHN will be a controlled Phase III study with a survival endpoint. In EU there might also be the option for an earlier approval based on PFS as endpoint based on an interim analysis. A decision on potential Rapporteur/Co-Rapporteur countries for the CP has not yet been taken. The choice will be based on the oncology expertise at the corresponding national EU authority. Another criteria could be an established working relationship between the pharmaceutical company and the authority. Based on the above mentioned criteria the EU authorities in Sweden, Germany, France, Netherlands or UK are potential candidates.

5.4.3.2 US

As stated above, the potential pivotal clinical trial in SCCHN will be a controlled Phase III study, likely with a survival endpoint. Given the indication and the high unmet medical need, it is anticipated that a successful trial will result in a full approval in the US. Assuming a successful designation as a fast track product, it is recommended that a 'rolling' submission will be used, whereby full portions of the application could be submitted for FDA review prior to submission of the complete dossier. This strategy could facilitate the priority review clock (which only starts counting upon receipt of the last piece of the dossier).

Details on the registration strategy and mechanisms applied would be determined during the End of Phase II meeting.

5.4.4 Marketing Authorization Strategy for Roll-out to Japan and to non-ICH-countries for the Monoclonal Antibody Monotuximab

As EU and USA are still the most important markets the preparation of the dossier will be first done for these two countries. As also other countries gets more and more important the preparations for the other countries should be initiated in parallel or shortly after the dossier preparation for EU and USA. Therefore a submission strategy for the roll-out to the other countries is initiated ideally already in the regulatory development plan or even during the preparation of dossier for the first MA submissions in EU and USA.

In the following the proposed submission strategy for roll-out to international (JP and non-ICH) countries for the developed mAb Monotuximab is presented.

The submission strategy is prepared based on own professional experiences and personal feedback from the different countries and regions (e.g. feedback received due to surveys made for the different countries and regions).

5.4.4.1 Registration Scenarios

5.4.4.1.1 Scenario 1: Early Stage Submission before Finalization of MA in EU and USA

This scenario covers the submission of the ICH dossier in Q3, 2011 as submitted in USA and in EU (via CP).

The dossier, which will be submitted in EU and USA in Q1, 2011, will be used for this scenario.

After finalization of the MA in USA and EU (e.g. in EU approx. in Q1, 2012, in USA maybe already in Q3/Q4, 2011), the updated global dossier (containing all changes which have to be done during the registration procedure (in EU changes in CP based on the questions by the CHMP)) and the EU/USA CPP will be submitted to the non-ICH DRAs. The submission of this updated dossier containing all changes made during the registration procedures in EU and USA will be necessary to bring these countries in line with the dossier as approved in EU and USA. As sometimes differences in the approved dossier between the US and EU are possible which cannot be implemented in one global dossier (or maybe also it is not desired to implement all changes requested from EU and US into the updated global dossier) it might happen that it has to be decided to use only the EU or the US approved dossier as basis for the updated global dossier for roll-out to international countries.

This strategy is the preferred one although it does not comply with most of the countries formal requirements (CPP of the intended Country of origin (CoO) for an authorized and marketed product). If it cannot be accepted at all (according to the estimation of local representatives in the different countries), the scenario as described in 5.4.4.1.2 will apply.

To summarize, the advantages of scenario 1 cover

- Early submission
- Necessity of updating the dossier after registration procedure only once resulting in reduced costs
- One global dossier for ensuring a high grade of compliance

5.4.4.1.2 Scenario 2: Submission after Finalization of MA in EU and USA

This scenario covers the use of the ICH dossier in Q2, 2012 as approved in EU and/or USA, with availability of the CPP for the MAA. It covers strictly the formal requirements of most of the non-ICH-countries.
An international submission of this dossier will be done with the EU/USA CPP, showing that the product is authorized (and marketed).
Summarizing, the advantages of this strategy cover
- The fact of availability of the EU/USA CPP
- No updates and therefore no costs for VARs
- One global dossier for ensuring a high grade of compliance
- A high level of formal acceptance by the countries

On the other hand, this strategy brings out a delay for submission of at least six months in comparison to scenario 1. Nevertheless, it is evident that a lot of countries will have to use this strategy.

5.4.4.2 Area Strategies
5.4.4.2.1 Asia

Based on experiences and surveys in the SEA countries regarding the acceptability of the above described scenarios revealed that many of the countries cannot accept to start with scenario 1 due to the missing ICH (EU and/or USA) approval and due to the necessity of the availability of the EU/USA CPP.
Therefore scenario 1 can be followed only in AUS, JP and South Korea.
Scenario 2 can be applied for China, Hong Kong, India, Indonesia, Malaysia, Philippines, Singapore, Taiwan, Thailand and Vietnam.
For JP no CPP is needed, so scenario 1 can be followed. In practice often additional activities and studies are needed, so that a submission in parallel or shortly after EU and USA is often not possible. Nevertheless if all prerequisites are fulfilled a parallel submission to EU and USA in JP is possible and should be taken into consideration (as JP is also a growing market with big market potential).

5.4.4.2.2 Latin America

In LA early stage submission as mentioned in scenario 1 is not possible in any country due to the missing EU/USA approval and the missing EU/USA CPP. Therefore scenario 2 will be used in all countries.
Countries, where scenario 2 has to be followed are Argentina, Brazil, Chile, Colombia, Costa Rica, Dominican Republic, Ecuador, El Salvador, Guatemala, Honduras, Mexico, Nicaragua, Panama, Peru, Uruguay and Venezuela.
Neither strategy 1 nor country specific strategies have to be applied for LA.

5.4.4.2.3 Middle East

In the ME countries the CPP from the CoO for an approved and marketed product is the basis for all registrations. In the case of a centrally authorized product also an EU CPP can be used. For Lebanon and Syria in addition to the EU CPP a CPP from the CoO have to be submitted with the MAA.
Consequently scenario 2 will be the general strategy for this area.
For Bahrain, Egypt, Kuwait, Iraq, Iran, Lebanon, Oman, Qatar, Saudi Arabia, Syria, United Arab Emirates and Yemen only scenario 2 can be used.

5.4.4.2.4 Switzerland, Eastern Europe, South Africa, Israel and Turkey

For CH no CPP is needed therefore scenario 1 will be followed. Submission can be done in parallel to EU and US and should be done if the necessary resources to do the submission are available. Otherwise submission will be done after approval in EU and USA.
For EE, South Africa, Israel and Turkey a survey regarding the necessity for a CPP has been made which revealed that most countries require a CPP from the CoO. For CP authorized products also the EU CPP is acceptable.
South Africa accepts any CPP and does not request a CPP at the time of submission: Scenario 1 will be followed and the EU/USA CPP - if requested - may be sent later.
Turkey and Russia do not request a CPP at the time of submission, therefore scenario 1 can be followed and the EU/USA CPP - if requested - may be sent later.
For Belarus, Croatia, Israel, Kazakhstan, Montenegro, Serbia and Ukraine scenario 2 has to be applied.

5.4.4.2.5 Africa

For AFR, the situation is quite complex due to the link of many African countries to a French MA and the French price. The Francophone African countries need the availability of the French MA as prerequisite for applying a MA in these countries. For the majority of countries it is necessary to wait for the availability of the French price for the product. The earliest submission for these countries will consequently be in Q2/Q3, 2012 (after the approval in EU and the pricing in France).
For Algeria and Tunisia scenario 2 has to be applied.
For Morocco, the prerequisite of the availability of the French price is not the case but the European approval including the availability of an EU CPP is needed to apply for a registration. Therefore also for Morocco scenario 2 applies.

5.4.4.3 "Master Dossier"

For Monotuximab it is recommended to implement a so-called "Master Dossier Concept".
The Master Dossier represents the most comprehensive information available on the product from a regulatory point of view. Ideally the first created Master Dossier is the submitted dossier in at least one key market, e.g. EU and/or USA. The Master Dossier consists of the complete structure and content of Modules 2, 3, 4, and 5 according to NtA. The Master Dossier is the basis of information to be used to generate the international Master Dossier for the non-ICH-countries.
After creation of the first Master Dossier (called Master 1 Dossier (M1 dossier)) which is the dossier submitted to EU and/or USA for the initial MAA of Monotuximab an updated Master Dossier will be created after the approval in EU and/or USA. This updated dossier is called Master 2 Dossier (M2 dossier). As the Master Dossier concept should be kept for the whole lifecycle of the product all updates and changed documentation submitted by VARs (e.g. applications for new indications) or REN to the EU and/or USA are included into the Master Dossier after approval in EU and/or USA. Such changes create an updated new version of the Master Dossier (next Master Dossier is then Master 3 (M3) Dossier).
Based on the full (complete) M1 and M2 dossiers containing all sections as submitted/ approved in EU/USA, so called international Master Dossiers (M1 int. and M2 int.) are created. These international Master Dossiers also contain Module 2, 3, 4 and 5. Compared to the ICH dossier, the highly confidential documents concerning DS section of Module 3 are shortened due to confidentiality reasons and IP issues. Therefore an international version of the DS section of Module 3 is created containing abbreviated

documents compared to the ICH dossier as the highly confidential information is deleted. The other documents of Module 2 and the complete Modules 4 and 5 are copied from the full ICH dossier and no documents are taken out for the international Master Dossier.

Additionally to Module 2 to 5, also some general sections of Module 1 (administrative information) like 1.4 Information about the Expert (Curriculum Vitae (CV) + expert signature pages), 1.6 Environmental Risk Assessment or 1.8 Information relating to Pharmacovigilance is recommend to be included in the Master Dossiers M1, M2 and M1 int. and M2 int. since it shall not be country specific.

5.4.4.4 Summary Table Concerning the Regulatory Strategy for the Marketing Authorization for the Different Countries

In the APPENDIX 20 a table summarizing the above described regulatory strategy for the different countries is provided. Within this table the registration scenario which is applicable, the dossier, which will be used for each country, the approx. timelines for sending out the dossier (assumed that all documents, studies, etc. for the countries are available) and the marketing priority (showing the market importance of the product within the different countries) is included. The table has the purpose to provide a short and compact overview on the regulatory strategy for MAA for ICH and non-ICH-countries.

5.5 Summary and Discussion

It is very important that the global development of a new substance (NBEs as well as NCEs) is based on the available ICH requirements as the ICH region is still the most important region for medicinal products based on market potential. In addition the growing markets like China, Brazil, Russia, India and ASEAN should be also kept in mind and the guidelines for these countries should be also carefully checked and be included in the global development program. If only the ICH requirements are included in the global development plan it might happen that additional studies like stability studies or preclinical studies or clinical studies needs to be created in order to be able to register the products in these non-ICH countries.

To be able to make a global development efficient and within quite short timelines a kind of global plan/route map including the main aspects of quality, preclinical and clinical strategy should be created. It is clear that all route maps/plans should be updated accordingly based on the status of development (please refer to APPENDIX 18).The whole regulatory development has to be done according to ICH guidelines and requirements in order to be able to get MAs in ICH region as well as in many non-ICH-countries as a lot of non-ICH countries following ICH requirements. In addition some national regulations and guidelines may be taken into consideration (e.g. stability requirements for ASEAN countries or some LA guidelines regarding stability for climatic zone III and IVA/IVB) in order to capture all needed requirements to be able to get MAs in all countries worldwide.

Within the CMC development plan the CMC development strategy is described which includes the objective of the CMC development program as well as the development strategy.

It is important to have the final formulation which is intended for submission of MAA ready before starting the Phase III trials. All guidelines and regulations with regard to stability requirements should be taken into consideration in order to be able to roll-out the MAA with all requested data to all countries worldwide as fast as possible. At the end of the plan there should be a decision tree to be able to decide for go/no go based on results of the proposed study program and short explanation for go/no go criteria should be provided.

This decision tree contains also so called "Decision points". One of these points is the decision to start the nonclinical development based on the results and the compound identified so far. If the results are promising the decision will be positive and the nonclinical development will be started. Based on experiences normally at the beginning of CMC development there are 100 compounds from which maybe 15-20 compounds (15-20%) will pass this first decision point and will go into nonclinical development. As mentioned before the final formulation of DP should be available before starting Phase III trials in order to perform the pivotal Phase III studies with the final formulation which will be then also submitted to apply for the MA. In case changes at the formulation during Phase III clinical studies are necessary these changes should be discussed with the authorities before submitting the changes in an IND amendment (USA) or CTA amendment (EU) to the authority.

In addition the following considerations should be taken into account during development of a new compound (NBE or NCE):

- Biomarker:
  - Biomarker should be included in clinical development phases
- Clinical issues and recommendations:
  - Perform Phase III studies according to ICH requirements (like randomized, uncontrolled, double-blind,...)
  - For some diseases registrations based on Phase II studies are possible (like for cancer indications)
  - In some countries for all diseases and indications mandatorily Phase III data needed (e.g. Brazil, Turkey) for getting a registration
  - Standard treatment for a disease might differ in the countries - therefore the comparison arm to the treatment arm has to be carefully selected
  - Some countries request local clinical trials like Vietnam, Taiwan, South Korea, China and Russia or they request participation in global trials with enough patients from their population
  - Pediatric studies (pediatric regulation - PIP/waiver)
  - Recommendation to perform two pivotal Phase III studies
  - Recommendation to include also Russia in global trials
  - Recommendation to include China in global trials with at least 200 patients (better 300 patients) in treatment arm

- Alternatively let China participates in global trial with less than 200 patients and do in addition a pan-Asian study with JP, China, Singapore Taiwan, South Korea, Vietnam and Hong Kong (as Vietnam, Taiwan and South Korea also request local clinical trials)
- CMC issues:
  - Stability data climatic zone III (30°C/35 % rh) and IV (IVA and IVB (30°C/75 % rh))
  - Requirements for two or more DS or DP manufacturers
- Administrative issues:
  - CPP availability
  - For most of the countries EU approval is prerequisite for submission and/or approval in the country

To provide a comprehensive overview of the requirements in the different regions worldwide for a new MAA please refer to requirements tables in APPENDIX 21.

During the last years the requirements for developing new medicinal products becomes more and more complex. Since some years it is e.g. mandatory to present also pediatric studies in EU and USA and also some other countries. These additional studies cost additional time and money for the companies. For some indications which do not occur in children it is possible to apply for a waiver in EU to avoid making studies in children. But for indications which have an incidence in children it is mandatory to make clinical trials in children before submitting the MAA. Also discussions whether to perform special clinical studies in elderly people are still ongoing and it has to be seen whether also such studies will become mandatory in future. Additionally there are more and more requirements to develop more patient tailored medicines which are more specific for special patient groups. One option to fulfill this goal is the usage of biomarkers. "*A biomarker (or a biological marker) is a substance which is used as an indicator for a biological status. A biomarker is characterized as it objectively measures and evaluates as an indicator for normal biological processes, pathogenic processes or pharmacologic responses to a therapeutic intervention. It is used in many scientific fields. For example in the medicinal field, a biomarker can be a substance whose detection indicates a particular disease state, for example, the presence of an antibody may indicate an infection. To make it more specific, a biomarker may indicate a change in expression or state of a protein that correlates with the risk or progression of a disease, or with the susceptibility of the disease to a given treatment. It can be also a substance that is introduced into an organism as a means to examine organ function or other aspects of health*".[60]

Therefore for newly developed medicinal products the authority is very keen on results on biomarkers to make the therapy more patient tailored. In many medicinal indications no approval will be possible any more without showing results on biomarkers. Therefore it is mandatory for the companies to include biomarkers into their development program for new medicinal products.

It is also very important to know that in some countries Phase II studies in general - independent of the indication of the medicinal product - are not sufficient for getting an approval for a MA. Therefore companies have to carefully plan their development concept and have to think whether to set up Phase III studies very early even in indications like cancer as a prerequisite to be able to get an approval in some countries like Brazil or Turkey. Otherwise the MA submission has to be postponed until the results of the Phase III trial are available. Also the comparison between the newly developed compound and the standard therapy might differ in the different countries. Therefore also the comparison arm to the treatment arm has to be carefully selected.

It is also recommended to perform two pivotal Phase III trials in one indication as the tendency can be observed that DRAs grant MA not always on results of one Phase III trial anymore. There is a risk for not getting a MA, especially if the results of the one pivotal Phase III trial are not outstanding.

Additionally some countries request mandatorily local clinical trials, e.g. in JP, Taiwan, South Korea, Vietnam, China or Russia or at least participation in global trials with enough patients. Enough patients in China e.g. mean that at least 200 patients minimum (better 300 patients) have to participate in the treatment arm! These numbers are mostly too high to be able to include so many patients of one population into a global trial (as there are also requirements how many Caucasian patients, etc. have to be included), therefore it is often not feasible to cover all requirements of the different countries by one global trial. As a consequence it is advisable to make in addition to the global trial so called regional trials, e.g. in Asia, or local trials in specific countries. As some Asian countries request a minimum number of patients participating in clinical trials it is possible to make a regional trial in Asian countries (so called pan-Asian study with JP, China, Singapore Taiwan, South Korea, Vietnam and Hong Kong) to fulfill all requests regarding clinical trials and to avoid making local clinical trials in the single countries.

---

[60] *http://en.wikipedia.org/wiki/Biomarker - dated 25.08.2010*

Not only the clinical aspects needs to be carefully evaluated for the global development there are also some CMC and administrative issues which needs to be taken into consideration. At least the requirements for stability data for climatic zone III (30°C/35 % rh) and IV (30°C/75 % rh) have to be considered and have to be fulfilled to be able to apply for a MA in countries which request stability data for climatic zone III and/or IV (e.g. Brazil). Without having these data a registration might be impossible or only possible with a very limited shelf-life as the available stability data for climatic zone I and II are not sufficient for these countries. Also in many countries it is not possible to have two or more manufacturers for DS or DP registered (e.g. in Taiwan, Brazil or Vietnam). These facts need to be taken also into consideration during the development.

Regarding administrative issues it is still today for many countries a prerequisite that companies have approval in EU and/or US before submitting a MA in the country. The CPP is a document showing that the product is approved in the country issuing the CPP and that the company is regularly inspected and is working according to GMP. The CPP is requested in many countries with submission of MA or at least during the evaluation process of the MA. Many countries until today will not grant a MA without the availability of a CPP. Countries where currently no CPP is needed for the approval of a MA are e.g. CH, AUS, Canada, South Korea and Russia.

In addition to the requirements for the dossier which needs to be submitted for getting a MA a lot of other aspects need to be carefully evaluated before and during the global development of a new compound. There are the marketing issues which are quite important to be kept in mind. It is important that marketing will evaluate quite early during the global development the market potential for the new compound in the indications which are under development by doing some market researches. A detailed marketing strategy for all indications under development needs to be developed for the new compound including the positioning against comparators. Also the observation and evaluation of competitors has to be done by marketing. Pricing is also an important issue for establishing the marketing strategy therefore the market research is very important to be able to evaluate which price can be established for the new medicinal product in which country. Pricing is a very sensitive issue as in many countries there are price limitations due to the governments. In additional the reimbursement issues need to be early evaluated whether the new medicinal product can be reimbursed in the different countries and which requirements need to be fulfilled to get the medicinal product reimbursed. It can be also anticipated that for future developments the proof of quality, safety and efficacy may not be sufficient but in addition the company has to proof also the cost benefit ratio for a new medicinal product by making some studies. Medicinal products which have shown a positive cost benefit ratio will be reimbursed. Besides the marketing aspects also a financial analysis has to be done including sales forecasts and net present value as well as the expected net present value. On the other hand also the research and development resources and costs, sales and marketing resources and costs and cost of goods have to be evaluated in order to calculate the approximately profit for the new medicinal product.

Also the IP situation is very important to be checked and evaluated. Normally if a new compound is under development the companies ask for a patent protection. The patent protection is valid for 20 years after its approval. As normally the global development of a new compound takes between 8 - 12 years the companies have only 8 - 12 years time left to earn money with the newly developed medicinal product. Therefore there is the possibility to apply in addition to the patent for a so called supplementary protection certificate (SPC) which can provide after patent expiry additional protection for maximum 5 years. So in total the company which develops a new compound can have patent protection and SPC protection in total for maximum 25 years. After expiry of these protections generic companies can come to the market.

In addition to patent protection in many countries there is also the possibility to get a data exclusivity. This means that if the applicant applies for a MA in this country the submitted dossier is protected for a certain time against generic companies. During the time of data exclusivity no generic company can make reference to the data of the originator company. In EU these data exclusivity period is 10 years, in US 5 years from day of approval of the MA. As normally the data exclusivity expires earlier than the patent it is possible for generic companies to submit after the expiry of data exclusivity (often also 2 years in advance of expiry of data exclusivity) and before patent expiry for the MA of the drug. The authorities will also grant the MA even the patent protection is still active. The generic company has then to wait for patent expiry before marketing its product, otherwise the patent holder can take legal steps against the generic company.

As in some countries the data exclusivity does not exist and the confidentiality of the submitted data are also sometimes not guaranteed the applicant has to think very carefully in which countries the MA dossier will be submitted and how many data will be presented to the authority. Besides that, the IP rights (like patent protection) are not yet established in all countries worldwide. So companies developing new compounds have to think quite early in development in which countries they would like to get MAs and in which countries they can and would like to apply for patents. As a patent has to be applied in each single country, which costs time and money for the company, the company has to think very carefully in which countries a patent protection is really useful and necessary.

So in summary, the companies developing new innovative medicinal products have to think about a lot of different issues during their development phases.
The changing environment for making global development of new products needs to be taken into consideration. Due to the political situation in many countries e.g. reforms of the health care systems (as many countries have to save money for their health care system) it becomes more and more difficult for the researching pharmaceutical companies to make global developments. In general, everybody would like to have new and innovative medicinal products better than the available drugs and especially for life threatening diseases but often people and the systems are not in favor to pay for these innovations. In many countries therefore the prices for new medicines are limited which means that companies have to think twice whether to introduce a new medicinal product into this market. Also the different markets are depending from each other - which means if a company would accept a certain price in one country (which is often lower than the price companies want to have for the medicinal product), other countries (e.g. neighbor countries) are looking for this price and make often an additional reduction of this price in their countries. E.g. the countries in ME region (like Saudi Arabia) ask for the reference prices in 30 countries (including EU countries, all neighbor countries in ME region) and based on the lowest price in these countries they will fix the price mostly again lower than the lowest price in the 30 requested countries. From a country perspective this makes sense in order to save money but for researching companies it unfortunately often leads to a situation that a drug will not be marketed in these countries as the price is too low to be rentable for the companies. As the development of a new medicinal products cost a lot of money and the patent protection of new medicinal products are limited (20 years patent protections plus 5 years protection through SPC) the companies need to have reinvested their development costs during these time. Therefore it is quite logical that new medicinal products are quite expensive and that the companies are not in favor to except all prices which countries offers them for their medicine. Therefore the tendency that certain drugs are not available in certain countries anymore because of price issues will probably increase during the next years. It has to be seen how governments in the countries and pharmaceutical companies will act and react on this issue which at the end goes to the expense of patients.

In principle the global submissions of an NBE or an NCE does not differ much regarding the submission strategy. In the past the development for NBEs and NCEs are mainly focused on EU and USA and consequently also the first submissions were prepared and done in EU and USA. Afterwards the other countries like JP, SEA, EE, LA, ME/AFR were covered. In future this will change certainly as pharmaceutical companies have recognized that also markets like JP, China or Russia become more and more importance. So in future the global submissions for NBEs or NCEs will not be focused first on EU and USA anymore but will also included countries like JP, China or Russia.

As mentioned before the main differences between the development and consequently also for the global submission strategy between an NBE and an NCE lie within the CMC part. Critical topics for NCEs are e.g. the definition of the starting materials or the analysis and characterization of the impurities. The critical topics regarding NBEs are the characterization and the manufacturing process. It is really strongly recommended to discuss such topics in advance with the DRAs. Another issue which often comes up during the submission of the MAA dossier in the different countries is the QC testing of the DS and DP. In many countries it is mandatorily requested to make at least a QC testing of the DP during or after the evaluation of the dossier. The evaluation of the dossier and the outcome of the QC testing is the basis for granting the MA in these countries. In case QC testing is requested the applicant has to provide DP, DS and if available also the impurities and/or degradation products of DP. The request for QC testing for NCEs is normally no issue for the applicants as the materials, equipment and expertise needed for performing the QC testing is mainly available at the DRAs and only the samples have to be provided. Sometimes - in case material and/or equipment are not available at the DRA laboratory - also material and/or equipment like HPLC columns are requested from the applicant. The applicant then provides the requested material and/or equipment and the DRA performs the QC testing. For NBEs the QC testing is often more complicated as some special materials and/or equipment are needed, e.g. for the testing of the biological activity often cells are needed. Besides the samples then also the missing materials like cells are requested from the applicant. As mentioned above the provision of samples should be also no issue for an NCE. But the provision of materials like cells is sometimes an issue as the cells are often patent protected (but not in all countries as patents don't exist in all countries or the applicant has not applied for the patent in all countries). One option to overcome these difficulties is the possibility to provide the cells accompanied with a confidentiality agreement which the DRA will sign and send back to the applicant. Within this confidentiality agreement the DRA guarantees that the cells are only used for the QC testing and are kept confidential. In many countries where no patent protection is available or not done by the applicant the DRAs are willing to sign such an agreement and to guarantee that the cells are only used for the QC testing.

After the QC testing is done and the evaluation of the dossier is finalized the MAA is granted. Should there be difficulties in performing the QC testing for an NBE or an NCE one possibility could be to invite the DRA to the laboratories of the applicant to demonstrate the QC testing.

Besides the differences in the CMC part there might be also a difference in the submission strategy regarding the sequence of submissions (e.g. in which countries the first submissions are made and the sequence of countries where the MAA will be submitted). Based on the expertise of the DRAs on NBEs or NCEs and on the indications for which the NBE or NCE is developed it might differ in which countries the first MAAs will be submitted. It is advisable to submit the MAA first in countries with a great experience and expertise on NBEs or NCEs as well as a great expertise in the developed indications to be able to get a registration quite fast. Dependent in which countries the first registrations are granted this might support the registration process also in other countries.

In summary it can be said that the only differences which can be seen regarding the submission strategy are regarding aspects in the CMC part and regarding the sequence of submissions (in which country to submit when the MAA dossier), otherwise there are not really differences in the submission strategy for an NBE or an NCE.

6 Conclusion and Outlook

This chapter describes the recommendation for development of a global regulatory strategy and provides a recommendation which regulatory procedure to use for which product. The recommendations are given based on my own experience in pharmaceutical industry for several years.

6.1 Recommendation which Regulatory Procedure to use for which Product

There are several regulatory aspects which have to be taken into account to decide which procedure (in case there are several regulatory procedures available in the countries) – should be used to apply for a MA in EU, USA, CADREAC, Singapore, China and Brazil.

In principle it is dependent on the kind of medicinal product which should be registered in the country. The different registration procedures have often well defined prerequisites under which circumstances which type of registration procedure can be used (please refer to the table " Comparison of different registration procedures in the different countries and pro/con arguments for each procedure" in chapter 4/page 90ff.) - so it is mostly not possible for the applicants to choose by themselves the type of registration procedure.

The accelerated procedures are in some countries only possible for MAAs of NCEs and not for NBEs due to the complexity of NBEs. In most countries fast track procedures are only applicable for serious or life-threatening diseases which have potential to address unmet medical need or for life-saving drugs or only for orphan drugs.

E.g. in EU for several kind of products the CP is mandatory so there is no choice of procedure (refer to section 3.2.2 and section 4), the same is also valid for other countries like CADREAC, China or USA. In Singapore it is dependent whether the medicinal product should be authorized before approval in the reference countries (like AUS, Canada, EU or USA) or whether to wait for submission until MA is granted in reference countries. In China there is also the possibility to apply for the MA before approval of the medicinal product in any country of the world via the special review procedure (see section 3.6.3 and section 4).

For using the accelerated procedures in the countries, there exists often very strict guidelines when and how to use these procedures.

The "normal" registration procedures are applicable for all kind of products and can be used by the applicant for all kind of MAAs.

Therefore it is advisable that the applicant evaluates very carefully before submission of an MAA which type of registration procedure can be used in which country for which type of product. In case of doubt or open questions it is advisable that the applicant may ask for a consultation meeting with the authority of the concerned country. After the registration procedures are chosen for each country the applicant can submit the MAA.

The different registration procedures in the countries have the identical main goal which is to protect human health and to make available new medicinal products as soon as possible. To evaluate the quality, safety and efficacy of the medicinal products is mandatory for getting approvals of the medicinal products.

To sum up, aspects like flexibility of the applicant/MAH, duration of the MA procedure, evaluation procedure of the dossier, date for submission of MAA, lifecycle of a product, harmonization of dossier and labeling documents (SPC and PIL), costs of the procedure and of course the product itself should be considered for the decision which procedure to be used for the MAA of a certain product in the different countries.

6.2 Recommendations for the Development of a Global Regulatory Strategy

In general, different regulations and procedures regarding the application for a new MA exist in the different countries worldwide. The main goal of all regulatory regulations and procedures in the countries are to protect human health by following them and to describe in details how to approve new safe medicinal products. Each medicinal product (NBE and NCEs) has to show highest quality, safety and efficacy.

The extent and the level of the requirements depend on the potential risk of harmful effects on human beings, animals and environment.

During the development of a new product (NBE or NCE) it is therefore mandatory to know all these regulations and requirements especially of the key markets where a submission of the dossier for the new product will be done after development. To identify the key markets for a new product the marketing divisions of a company will evaluate during the development phases the market potential of the new product (NBE and NCE) under development. Based on this market research the whole global development program will be established with the goal to get registration as fast as possible in the key markets. Within the global development program all aspects concerning quality, safety and efficacy based on the current available legislations (regulations, directives and guidelines) have to be incorporated. It is advisable to create a global development team. This global development team should consist at least of representatives from the following functions: one representative from CMC, one representative from nonclinical (maybe one from toxicology and one from pharmacology), one representative from clinical, one representative from regulatory affairs and one representative from marketing. In addition the team should be led from a global development team leader and should have also one project manager as member for all project coordinating work. The adequate time point for creation of such a global development team is after finalization of Phase 0 - before starting with clinical trials.

It is emphasized that it is strongly recommended to include a representative from regulatory affairs in the global development team beginning latest after Phase 0 (latest after the nonclinical development is done). For the whole further development of a new compound the regulatory advice should be provided especially with regard to guidelines, regulations, etc. This is true for the CMC development as well as for the clinical development. The regulatory affairs representative can provide advice how to set up a clinical trial with regard to current regulation and guidelines to ensure that the clinical trial is performed according to the current regulations and guidelines. Otherwise there is the risk that the authority won't accept the trial if it is not performed according to current regulations and guidelines. This risk normally no company would like to take as especially the clinical development is quite expensive during the development of a new compound.

In general it is advisable that the global team is the decision making board for the new product under development. For the most important decisions which are mostly also the most cost intensive decisions (like go on from Phase II to Phase III) it is mandatory that the global team will make a recommendation based on the available data and the upper management will decide finally.

During the last years the requirements for developing new medicinal products becomes more and more complex. Since some years it is e.g. mandatory to present also pediatric studies in EU and USA and also in some other countries. These additional studies cost additional time and money for the companies. For some indications which are not available in children it is possible to apply for a waiver in EU to avoid making studies in children. But for indications which are also available in children it is mandatory to make clinical trials in children before submitting the MAA. Also discussions whether special clinical studies in the elderly are still ongoing and it has to be seen whether also such studies become mandatory in future.

The highest goal for the development of new compounds for sure is the safety of the patients and also the proof of efficacy of the new medicinal product. For these goals the companies are surely willing to invest a lot of money to develop new innovative safe and efficient medicinal product. On the other hand the companies also need to have a return of investment (they should earn at least the money they invested in the development of the product). If in future companies have to recognize that there is no return of investment any more due to health economic issues like price reductions there might come the day where companies are not willing to develop new medicinal products any more as the development of new products costs more money that it brings back. Therefore the politicians in the different countries should evaluate very carefully the health care system before doing some reforms which at the end might be a disadvantage for the patients because of the non availability of innovative drugs any more.

Regarding this issue especially the changing environment for making global development of new products needs to be taken into consideration. Due to the political situation in many countries e.g. reforms of the health care systems it becomes more and more difficult for researching pharmaceutical companies to make global development. In principle everybody would like to have new and innovative medicinal products especially against life threatening diseases but often the people and the systems are not in favor to pay for these innovations. In many countries therefore the prices for new medicines are limited which means that companies have to think twice whether to introduce a new medicinal product into this market. As the development of a new medicinal products cost a lot of money and the patent protection of new medicinal products are limited (20 years patent protections plus 5 years protection through supplementary protection certificate (SPC)) companies should have reinvested their development costs during these protected time. Therefore it is quite logical that new medicinal products are quite expensive.

All discussed issues and recommendations should be taken into consideration for future developments.

In the past the focus in development lies clearly on the ICH region, mainly EU and USA. Companies make the global development based on these two markets (EU and USA). The development for other countries often started after the initial approval in EU and/or USA. This led often to a situation that approval in countries outside ICH can be achieved only years after the initial approvals in EU and USA as additional studies (like special stability studies, pharmacodynamic (PD) and/or pharmacokinetic (PK) studies or clinical studies) are needed for these countries. As countries outside ICH will become more and more important from their market potential companies are interested to receive approvals in these countries as early as possible. Therefore the global development of a new product should not be focused any more only on EU and USA in the first step. Countries like China, Russia, Brazil or India should be included in the global development quite early to be able to make parallel submissions or at least to submit as soon as an approval in EU and/or US is achieved.

Based on the already discussed issues it can be anticipated that it will get more difficult to get new medicinal products approved in future. The requirements to get a medicinal product approved increase compared to some years ago and it might happen that the requirements will increase further. During the last years the tendency can be observed that more patient tailored drugs are requested by authorities compared to products approved in very broad indications. Companies are requested to develop patient tailored drugs. This might be not so beneficial from a company perspective as the number of patients which can be treated with one medicinal product which is patient tailored might be smaller. Nevertheless, this is the direction agencies might follow in future. Therefore topics like biomarkers or other specific markers to identify patient tailored drugs will become more and more important in future. It is advisable for companies to include biomarkers or other specific marker in their development program of a new compound as otherwise authorities might not grant the submitted MA. In order to be sure what authorities want it is recommended to make scientific meetings with the authorities to discuss and agree on the clinical development program especially with regard to setting of clinical trials, endpoints and biomarkers/specific markers.

Due to the higher requirements for developing new compounds also the development time and costs might increase. Therefore companies are interested to get high prices for new medicinal products in order to get their return on investment during the running patent period and data exclusivity period back to be able to invest the earned money in the development of other new compounds.

Also other aspects like health economic aspects will become more and more important. Currently in many countries companies are free in setting the prices for new medicinal products which are normally quite high. If the medicinal product is reimbursed in a country the health care system has to pay the high price for the medicinal product. As many health care systems are not able to pay so many money anymore in future it is most likely that governments will limit prices for new medicinal products in many countries in order to relieve the health care systems. It can be also anticipated that for future developments the proof of quality, safety and efficacy may not be sufficient but in addition the company has to proof also the cost benefit ratio for a new medicinal product by making some studies. Medicinal products which have shown a positive cost benefit ratio will be reimbursed. This might lead to the situation that companies will not register and marketed new medicinal products in all countries in future as the price offered to get for the new medicinal product might be too low. This is a bad situation for patients as they might not be able to receive new drugs in future although the need for innovative new medicinal products will exceed especially due to the excess of age in the population.

In conclusion the requirements to get a drug registered and reimbursed will increase and consequently the development costs for companies will increase, too. It has to be awaited how government will build up the health care systems in future and how requirements will change. One possible solution to deal with the increase costs for development and the increasing requirements might be that pharmaceutical companies will merge and will develop new innovative medicinal products together and share the development costs. This will be especially attractive for small and medium-sized companies. Also companies might think about the location of their development centers in order to optimize the development. It is recommended that companies will have only one or two global development centers where the global development for all new compounds is done.

Companies can also think about an "award" for fast and goal oriented development of new drugs. This might be an additional motivation for co-workers to work more efficient and to fasten the development of new drugs.

Pharmaceutical companies should be in close contact with authorities in order to be able to fulfill all requirements needed to get a new medicinal product approved and marketed. Companies should be also in close contacts with governments and health care systems in order to fulfill their requirements and in order to be able to influence them with regard to decisions on health care systems.

Authorities and governments should offer pharmaceutical companies some incentives in order to advance the development of new innovative drugs.

As the requirements increase for getting new drugs registered, authorities might offer an incentive for companies developing new innovative drugs in future. Such incentives could be e.g. a longer data exclusivity period (as protection against generic companies), market exclusivity for some additional years or reduction of registration costs.

Besides all increasing barriers for getting new products approved and marketed, it is of utmost importance that the development of new innovative medicinal product will be continued to offer patients best medicinal supply.

Therefore it seems to be logical that pharmaceutical companies, authorities and governments have to work together and find solutions that the development of new innovative drugs will be attractive and efficient for all sites in future.

7 Preliminary Publications and Presentations

Hörner A. "Describe the CADREAC-procedure for a product which was authorized via mutual recognition procedure in the EU and compare the CADREAC-procedure with the national procedure in one CADREAC country (e.g. Romania)", Wissenschaftliche Prüfungsarbeit zur Erlangung des Titels „Master of Drug Regulatory Affairs" der Mathematisch-Naturwissenschaftlichen Fakultät der Rheinischen Friedrich-Wilhelms-Universität Bonn, May 2005; available from http://www.dgra.de/studiengang/master_thesis/hoerner.php and http://www.dgra.de/studiengang/pdf/master_hoerner_a.pdf, accessed August 6, 2010

Hörner A. "Analysis of requirements for a new marketing authorization application for new chemical entities and new biological entities" Doktoranden-Vortragstag. Bonn: Rheinische Friedrich-Wilhelms-Universität Bonn, April 04, 2008; available from http://home.arcor.de/janna-schweim/8-Hoerner.pdf, accessed August 6, 2010

Hörner A. "General requirements for a new marketing authorization application with focus on ASEAN" Doktoranden-Vortragstag Bonn: Rheinische Friedrich-Wilhelms-Universität Bonn, April 25, 2009; available from http://www.harald-g-schweim.de/Hoerner-2009.pdf; Internet; accessed August 6, 2010

Herrmann A. "General information, drug development and requirements for a new marketing authorization application for new chemical entities and new biological entities in China" Doktoranden-Vortragstag. Bonn: Rheinische Friedrich-Wilhelms-Universität Bonn, May 29, 2010; available from http://www.harald-schweim.de/09-Herrmann-2010.pdf Internet; accessed August 6, 2010.

Herrmann A., Schweim H.G. "The Benefits of Joining nCADREAC" in Regulatory Affairs Journal (RAJ) Pharma, August 2010, P-485-487

8 Appendices

APPENDIX 1 CTD TABLE OF CONTENTS

The table of contents (ToCs) of Module 2 – 5 of the ICH CTD dossier is enclosed as an attachment:

- **Module 2: CTD Summaries**

  Module 2.1 CTD ToCs (Module 2 – 5)

  Module 2.2 Introduction

  Module 2.3 Quality Overall Summary (QOS)

  Module 2.4 Nonclinical Overview (NCO)

  Module 2.5 Clinical Overview (CO)

  Module 2.6 Nonclinical Summary

  Module 2.7 Clinical Summary

- **Module 3: Quality - Chemical-pharmaceutical and biological information for chemical active substances and biological medicinal product**

  3.1 Module 3 ToC

  3.2 Body of data

  3.2.S Drug substance (DS)

  3.2.S.1 General Information

  3.2.S.1.1 Nomenclature

  3.2.S.1.2 Structure

  3.2.S.1.3 General properties

  3.2.S.2 Manufacture

  3.2.S.2.1 Manufacturer(s)

  3.2.S.2.2 Description of manufacturing process and process controls

  3.2.S.2.3 Control of materials

  3.2.S.2.4 Controls of critical steps and intermediates (Biotech)

  3.2.S.2.5 Process validation and or evaluation

  3.2.S.2.6 Manufacturing process development

  3.2.S.3 Characterization

  3.2.S.3.1 Elucidation of structure and other characteristics

  3.2.S.3.2 Impurities

  3.2.S.4 Control of drug substance

  3.2.S.4.1 Specification

  3.2.S.4.2 Analytical procedures

3.2.S.4.3 Validation of analytical procedures

3.2.S.4.4 Batch analyses

3.2.S.4.5 Justification of specifications

3.2.S.5 Reference standards of materials

3.2.S.6 Container closure system

3.2.S.7 Stability

3.2.S.7.1 Stability summary and conclusions

3.2.S.7.2 Post-approval stability protocol and stability commitment

3.2.S.7.3 Stability data

3.2.P Drug product (DP)

3.2.P.1 Description and composition of the drug product

3.2.P.2 Pharmaceutical development

3.2.P.3 Manufacture

3.2.P.3.1 Manufacturer(s)

3.2.P.3.2 Batch formula

3.2.P.3.3 Description of manufacturing process and process controls

3.2.P.3.4 Controls of critical steps and intermediates

3.2.P.3.5 Process validation and or evaluation

3.2.P.4 Control of excipients

3.2.P.4.1 Specifications

3.2.P.4.2 Analytical procedures

3.2.P.4.3 Validation of analytical procedures

3.2.P.4.4 Justification of specifications

3.2.P.4.5 Excipients of human or animal origin

3.2.P.4.6 Novel excipients

3.2.P.5 Control of drug product

3.2.P.5.1 Specifications

3.2.P.5.2 Analytical procedures

3.2.P.5.3 Validation of analytical procedures

3.2.P.5.4 Batch analyses

3.2.P.5.5 Characterization of impurities

3.2.P.5.6 Justification of specifications

3.2.P.6 Reference standards or materials

3.2.P.7 Container closure system

3.2.P.8 Stability
3.2.P.8.1 Stability summary and conclusion
3.2.P.8.2 Post-approval stability protocol and stability commitment

3.2.P.8.3 Stability data

3.2.A Appendices
3.2.A.1 Facilities and equipment
3.2.A.2 Adventitious agents safety evaluation
3.2.A.3 Novel excipients
3.2.R Regional information
3.2.R.1 Batch records
3.2.R.2 Process validation scheme for the drug product
3.2.R.3 Medical device
3.2.R.4 Medicinal products containing or using in the manufacturing process materials of animal and/or human origin

3.3 Literature references

- **Module 4: Nonclinical Study Reports**
  4.1 ToCs of Module 4
  4.2 Study Reports
  4.2.1 Pharmacology
  4.2.1.1 Primary Pharmacodynamics
  4.2.1.2 Secondary Pharmacodynamics
  4.2.1.3 Safety Pharmacology
  4.2.1.4 Pharmacodynamic Drug Interactions
  4.2.2 Pharmacokinetics
  4.2.2.1 Analytical Methods and Validation Reports (if separate reports are available)
  4.2.2.2 Absorption
  4.2.2.3 Distribution
  4.2.2.4 Metabolism
  4.2.2.5 Excretion
  4.2.2.6 Pharmacokinetic Drug Interactions (nonclinical)
  4.2.2.7 Other Pharmacokinetic Studies

4.2.3 Toxicology

4.2.3.1 Single-Dose Toxicity (in order by species, by route)

4.2.3.2 Repeat-Dose Toxicity (in order by species, by route, by duration; including supportive toxicokinetics evaluations)

4.2.3.3 Genotoxicity

4.2.3.3.1 In vitro

4.2.3.3.2 In vivo (including supportive toxicokinetics evaluations)

4.2.3.4 Carcinogenicity (including supportive toxicokinetics evaluations)

4.2.3.4.1 Long-term studies (in order by species; including range finding studies that cannot appropriately be included under repeat-dose toxicity or pharmacokinetics)

4.2.3.4.2 Short- or medium-term studies (including range-finding studies that cannot appropriately be included under repeat dose toxicity or pharmacokinetics)

4.2.3.4.3 Other studies

4.2.3.5 Reproductive and Developmental Toxicity (including range-finding studies and supportive toxicokinetics evaluations) (If modified study designs are used, the following sub-headings should be modified accordingly.)

4.2.3.5.1 Fertility and early embryonic development

4.2.3.5.2 Embryo-fetal development

4.2.3.5.3 Prenatal and postnatal development, including maternal function

4.2.3.5.4 Studies in which the offspring (juvenile animals) are dosed and/or further evaluated.

4.2.3.6 Local Tolerance

4.2.3.7 Other Toxicity Studies (if available)

4.2.3.7.1 Antigenicity

4.2.3.7.2 Immunotoxicity

4.2.3.7.3 Mechanistic studies (if not included elsewhere)

4.2.3.7.4 Dependence

4.2.3.7.5 Metabolites

4.2.3.7.6 Impurities

4.2.3.7.7 Other

4.3 Literature references

♦ **Module 5: Clinical Study Reports**
5.1 ToCs of Module 5
5.2 Tabular Listing of All Clinical Studies
5.3 Clinical Study Reports
5.3.1 Reports of Biopharmaceutic Studies
5.3.1.1 Bioavailability (BA) Study Reports
5.3.1.2 Comparative BA and Bioequivalence (BE) Study Reports
5.3.1.3 In vitro-In vivo Correlation Study Reports
5.3.1.4 Reports of Bioanalytical and Analytical Methods for Human Studies
5.3.2 Reports of Studies Pertinent to Pharmacokinetics using Human Biomaterials
5.3.2.1 Plasma Protein Binding Study Reports
5.3.2.2 Reports of Hepatic Metabolism and Drug Interaction Studies
5.3.2.3 Reports of Studies Using Other Human Biomaterials
5.3.3 Reports of Human Pharmacokinetic (PK) Studies
5.3.3.1 Healthy Subject PK and Initial Tolerability Study Reports
5.3.3.2 Patient PK and Initial Tolerability Study Reports
5.3.3.3 Intrinsic Factor PK Study Reports
5.3.3.4 Extrinsic Factor PK Study Reports
5.3.3.5 Population PK Study Reports
5.3.4 Reports of Human Pharmacodynamic (PD) Studies
5.3.4.1 Healthy Subject PD and PK/PD Study Reports
5.3.4.2 Patient PD and PK/PD Study Reports
5.3.5 Reports of Efficacy and Safety Studies
5.3.5.1 Study Reports of Controlled Clinical Studies Pertinent to the Claimed Indication
5.3.5.2 Study Reports of Uncontrolled Clinical Studies
5.3.5.3 Reports of Analyses of Data from More Than One Study
5.3.5.4 Other Clinical Study Reports
5.3.6 Reports of Post-Marketing Experience
5.3.7 Case Report Forms and Individual Patient Listings

5.4 Literature References

APPENDIX 2   CTD TABLE OF CONTENT FOR EU MODULE 1

♦ Module 1: Administrative Information and Prescribing Information

Table of Content

1.0 Cover Letter

1.1 Comprehensive Table of Contents

1.2 Application Form

1.3 Product Information

1.3.1 Summary of product characteristics (SPC), Labeling and Package Leaflet (PIL)

1.3.2 Mock-up

1.3.3 Specimen

1.3.4 Consultation with Target Patient Groups

1.3.5 Product Information already approved in the Member States

1.3.6 Braille

1.4 Information about the Experts

1.4.1 Quality

1.4.2 Non-Clinical

1.4.3 Clinical

1.5 Specific Requirements for Different Types of Applications

1.5.1 Information for Bibliographical Applications

1.5.2 Information for Generic, 'Hybrid' or Bio-similar Applications

1.5.3 (Extended) Data/Market Exclusivity

1.5.4 Exceptional Circumstances

1.5.5 Conditional Marketing Authorisation

1.6 Environmental Risk Assessment

1.6.1 Non-GMO

1.6.2 GMO

1.7 Information relating to Orphan Market Exclusivity

1.7.1 Similarity

1.7.2 Market Exclusivity

1.8 Information relating to Pharmacovigilance

1.8.1 Pharmacovigilance System

1.8.2 Risk-management System

1.9 Information relating to Clinical Trials

Responses to Questions

Additional Data

APPENDIX 3 DIFFERENCES NBE AND NCE WITH REGARD TO MODULE 2 AND 3

For detailed information please refer to the attached table[12]

	NCE	NBE
Module 2 Section: 2.3.S.3 Characterization (name, manufacturer)	A summary of the interpretation of evidence of structure and isomerism, as described in 3.2.S.3.1, should be included. When a drug substance is chiral, it should be specified whether specific stereoisomers or a mixture of stereoisomers have been used in the nonclinical and clinical studies, and information should be given as to the stereoisomer of the drug substance that is to be used in the final product intended for marketing. For NCE and Biotech: The QOS should summarize the data on potential and actual impurities arising from the synthesis, manufacture and/or degradation, and should summarize the basis for setting the acceptance criteria for individual and total impurities. The QOS should also summarize the impurity levels in batches of the drug substance used in the non-clinical studies, in the clinical trials, and in typical batches manufactured by the proposed commercial process. The QOS should state how the proposed impurity limits are qualified. *A tabulated summary of the data provided in 3.2.S.3.2, with graphical representation, where appropriate should be included.*	For Biotech: A description of the desired product and product-related substances and a summary of general properties, characteristic features and characterization data (for example, primary and higher order structure and biological activity), as described in 3.2.S.3.1, should be included.

	NCE	NBE
Module 3 3.2.S.1.2 Structure (name, manufacturer)	NCE: The structural formula, including relative and absolute stereochemistry, the molecular formula, and the relative molecular mass should be provided. Reference CPMP-Guidelines: "Chemistry of the New Active Substance" and "Chemistry of the Active Substance"	Biotech: The schematic amino acid sequence indicating glycosylation sites or other posttranslational modifications and relative molecular mass should be provided, as appropriate. Reference CPMP Guidelines: "Chemistry of the New Active Substance" and "Chemistry of the Active Substance"
Module 3 3.2.S.2.2 Description of Manufacturing Process and Process Controls (name, manufacturer)	NCE: A flow diagram of the synthetic process(es) should be provided that includes molecular formulae, weights, yield ranges, chemical structures of starting materials, intermediates, reagents and drug substance reflecting stereochemistry, and identifies operating conditions and solvents. A sequential procedural narrative of the manufacturing process should be submitted. The narrative should include, for example, quantities of raw materials, solvents, catalysts and reagents reflecting the representative batch scale for commercial manufacture, identification of critical steps, process controls, equipment and operating conditions (e.g., temperature, pressure, pH, time). Alternate processes should be explained and described with the same level of detail as the primary process. Reprocessing steps should be identified and justified. Any data to support this justification should be either referenced or filed in	Biotech: Information should be provided on the manufacturing process, which typically starts with a vial(s) of the cell bank, and includes cell culture, harvest(s), purification and modification reactions, filling, storage and shipping conditions. Batch(es) and scale definition. An explanation of the batch numbering system, including information regarding any pooling of harvests or intermediates and batch size or scale should be provided. Cell culture and harvest. A flow diagram should be provided that illustrates the manufacturing route from the original inoculum (e.g. cells contained in one or more vials(s) of the Working Cell Bank up to the last harvesting operation. The diagram should include all steps (i.e., unit operations) and intermediates. Relevant information for each stage, such as population doubling levels, cell concentration, volumes, pH, cultivation times, holding times, and temperature, should be included. Critical steps and critical intermediates for which specifications are established (as mentioned in 3.2.S.2.4) should be identified.

	NCE	NBE
	3.2.S.2.5.	A description of each process step in the flow diagram should be provided. Information should be included on, for example, scale; culture media and other additives (details provided in 3.2.S.2.3); major equipment (details provided in 3.2.A.1); and process controls, including in-process tests and operational parameters, process steps, equipment and intermediates with acceptance criteria (details provided in 3.2.S.2.4). Information on procedures used to transfer material between steps, equipment, areas, and buildings, as appropriate, and shipping and storage conditions should be provided. (Details on shipping and storage provided in 3.2.S.2.4.). Purification and modification reactions A flow diagram should be provided that illustrates the purification steps (i.e., unit operations) from the crude harvest(s) up to the step preceding filling of the drug substance. All steps and intermediates and relevant information for each stage (e.g., volumes, pH, critical processing time, holding times, temperatures and elution profiles and selection of fraction, storage of intermediate, if applicable) should be included. Critical steps for which specifications are established as mentioned in 3.2.S.2.4 should be identified. A description of each process step (as identified in the flow diagram) should be provided. The description should include information on, for example, scale, buffers and other reagents (details provided in 3.2.S.2.3, major equipment (details provided in 3.2.A.1), and materials. For materials such as membranes

	NCE	NBE
		and chromatography resins, information for conditions of use and reuse also should be provided. (Equipment details in 3.2.A.1; validation studies for the reuse and regeneration of columns and membranes in 3.2.S.2.5.) The description should include process controls (including in-process tests and operational parameters) with acceptance criteria for process steps, equipment and intermediates. (Details in 3.2.S.2.4.).
		Reprocessing procedures with criteria for reprocessing of any intermediate or the drug substance should be described. (Details should be given in 3.2.S.2.5.).
		Information on procedures used to transfer material between steps, equipment, areas, and buildings, as appropriate, and shipping and storage conditions should be provided (details on shipping and storage provided in 3.2.S.2.4.).
		Filling, storage and transportation (shipping)
		A description of the filling procedure for the drug substance, process controls (including in-process tests and operational parameters), and acceptance criteria should be provided. (Details in 3.2.S.2.4.) The container closure system(s) used for storage of the drug substance (details in 3.2.S.6.) and storage and shipping conditions for the drug substance should be described.
Module 3	NCEs and Biotech:	Biotech:
3.2.S.2.3 Control of Materials (name, manufacturer)	Materials used in the manufacture of the drug substance (e.g., raw materials, starting materials, solvents, reagents, catalysts) should be listed identifying	Materials used in the manufacture of the drug substance (e.g., raw materials, starting materials, solvents, reagents, catalysts) should be listed identifying where each material is used in the

	NCE	NBE
	where each material is used in the process. Information on the quality and control of these materials should be provided. Information demonstrating that materials (including biologically-sourced materials, e.g., media components, monoclonal antibodies, enzymes) meet standards appropriate for their intended use (including the clearance or control of adventitious agents) should be provided, as appropriate. For biologically-sourced materials, this can include information regarding the source, manufacture, and characterization. (Details in 3.2.A.2 for both NCE and Biotech)	process. Information on the quality and control of these materials should be provided. Information demonstrating that materials (including biologically-sourced materials, e.g., media components, monoclonal antibodies, enzymes) meet standards appropriate for their intended use (including the clearance or control of adventitious agents) should be provided, as appropriate. For biologically-sourced materials, this can include information regarding the source, manufacture, and characterization. (Details in 3.2.A.2 for both NCE and Biotech)
		Additional for Biotech:
		Control of Source and Starting Materials of Biological Origin
		Summaries of viral safety information for biologically-sourced materials should be provided. (Details in 3.2.A.2.)
		Source, history, and generation of the cell substrate
		Information on the source of the cell substrate and analysis of the expression construct used to genetically modify cells and incorporated in the initial cell clone used to develop the Master Cell Bank should be provided as described in CPMPICH Guidelines Q5B and Q5D.
		Cell banking system, characterization, and testing
		Information on the cell banking system, quality control activities, and cell line stability during production and storage (including procedures used to generate the Master and Working Cell Bank(s)) should be provided as described in CPMP-ICH Guidelines Q5B and Q5D.

	NCE	NBE
Module 3 **3.2.S.2.5 Process Validation and/or Evaluation (name, manufacturer)**	Process validation and/or evaluation studies for aseptic processing and sterilization should be included.	Process validation and/or evaluation studies for aseptic processing and sterilization should be included. **Biotech:** Sufficient information should be provided on validation and evaluation studies to demonstrate that the manufacturing process (including reprocessing steps) is suitable for its intended purpose and to substantiate selection of critical process controls (operational parameters and in-process tests) and their limits for critical manufacturing steps (e.g., cell culture, harvesting, purification, and modification). The plan for conducting the study should be described and the results, analysis and conclusions from the executed study(ies) should be provided. The analytical procedures and corresponding validation should be cross-referenced (e.g., 3.2.S.2.4, 3.2.S.4.3) or provided as part of justifying the selection of critical process controls and acceptance criteria. For manufacturing steps intended to remove or inactivate viral contaminants, the information from evaluation studies should be provided in 3.2.A.2.
Module 3 **3.2.S.2.6 Manufacturing Process Development (name, manufacturer)**	**NCE:** A description and discussion should be provided of the significant changes made to the manufacturing process and/or manufacturing site of the drug substance used in producing nonclinical, clinical, scale-up, pilot, and, if available, production scale batches. Reference should be made to the drug substance data	**Biotech:** The developmental history of the manufacturing process, as described in 3.2.S.2.2, should be provided. The description of change(s) made to the manufacture of drug substance batches used in support of the marketing application (e.g., nonclinical or clinical studies) should include, for example, changes to the process or to critical equipment. The reason for the change should be explained. Relevant information on drug

	NCE	NBE
	provided in section 3.2.S.4.4. Reference CPMP-ICH Guideline: "Impurities testing guideline: impurities in new drug substances	substance batches manufactured during development, such as the batch number, manufacturing scale, and use (e.g., stability, nonclinical, reference material) in relation to the change, should be provided. The significance of the change should be assessed by evaluating its potential to impact the quality of the drug substance (and/or intermediate, if appropriate). For manufacturing changes that are considered significant, data from comparative analytical testing on relevant drug substance batches should be provided to determine the impact on quality of the drug substance (see Q6B for additional guidance). A discussion of the data, including a justification for selection of the tests and assessment of results, should be included. Testing used to assess the impact of manufacturing changes on the drug substance(s) and the corresponding drug product(s) can also include nonclinical and clinical studies. Cross-reference to the location of these studies in other modules of the submission should be included. Reference should be made to the drug substance data provided in section 3.2.S.4.4.
Module 3 3.2.S.3 Characterization (name, manufacturer) 3.2.S.3.1 Elucidation of Structure and other Characteristics (name, manufacturer)	NCE: Confirmation of structure based on e.g., synthetic route and spectral analyses should be provided. Information such as the potential for isomerism, the identification of stereochemistry, or the potential for forming polymorphs should also be included.	Biotech: For desired product and product-related substances, details should be provided on primary, secondary and higher-order structure, post-translational forms (e.g., glycoforms), biological activity, purity, and immunochemical properties, when relevant.

	NCE	NBE
Module 3 3.2.A APPENDICES 3.2.A.1 Facilities and Equipment (name, manufacturer) Biotech:		Biotech: A diagram should be provided illustrating the manufacturing flow including movement of raw materials, personnel, waste, and intermediate(s) in and out of the manufacturing areas. Information should be presented with respect to adjacent areas or rooms that may be of concern for maintaining integrity of the product. Information on all developmental or approved products manufactured or manipulated in the same areas as the applicant's product should be included. A summary description of product-contact equipment, and its use (dedicated or multi-use) should be provided. Information on preparation, cleaning, sterilization, and storage of specified equipment and materials should be included, as appropriate. Information should be included on procedures (e.g., cleaning and production scheduling) and design features of the facility (e.g., area classifications) to prevent contamination or cross-contamination of areas and equipment, where operations for the preparation of cell banks and product manufacturing are performed.
Module 3 3.2.A.2 Adventitious Agents Safety Evaluation (name, dosage form, manufacturer)		Information assessing the risk with respect to potential contamination with adventitious agents should be provided in this section. **For non-viral adventitious agents:** Detailed information should be provided on the avoidance and control of non-viral adventitious agents (e.g., transmissible spongiform encephalopathy agents, bacteria, mycoplasma, fungi). This information can include, for example, certification

NCE	NBE
	and/or testing of raw materials and excipients, and control of the production process, as appropriate for the material, process and agent.

Reference CPMP-ICH Guidelines: "Derivation and Characterization of Cell Substrates Used for Production of Biotechnological/ Biological Products", "Specifications: Test Procedures and Acceptance Criteria for Biotechnological/ Biological Products"

Reference CPMP Guideline: "Minimizing the Risk of Transmitting animal Spongiform Encephalopathy Agents via Medicinal Products"

For viral adventitious agents:

Detailed information from viral safety evaluation studies should be provided in this section. Viral evaluation studies should demonstrate that the materials used in production are considered safe, and that the approaches used to test, evaluate, and eliminate the potential risks during manufacturing are suitable.

Reference CPMP-ICH Guidelines: "Viral Safety Evaluation of Biotechnology Products Derived From Cell Lines of Human or Animal Origin", "Derivation and Characterization of Cell Substrates Used for Production of Biotechnological/ Biological Products", "Specifications: Test Procedures and Acceptance Criteria for Biotechnological/ Biological Products" Reference CPMP Guideline: " virus validation studies: the design, contribution and interpretation of studies validating the inactivation and removal of viruses"

Materials of Biological Origin

Information essential to evaluate the virological safety of materials of animal or human origin (e.g. |

NCE	NBE
	biological fluids, tissue, organ, cell lines) should be provided. (See related information in 3.2.S.2.3, and 3.2.P.4.5). For cell lines, information on the selection, testing, and safety assessment for potential viral contamination of the cells and viral qualification of cell banks should also be provided. (See related information in 3.2.S.2.3). Testing at appropriate stages of production The selection of virological tests that are conducted during manufacturing (e.g., cell substrate, unprocessed bulk or post viral clearance testing) should be justified. The type of test, sensitivity and specificity of the test, if applicable, and frequency of testing should be included. Test results to confirm, at an appropriate stage of manufacture, that the product is free from viral contamination should be provided. (See related information in 3.2.S.2.4 and 3.2.P.3.4). Viral Testing of Unprocessed Bulk In accordance with Q5A and Q6B, results for viral testing of unprocessed bulk should be included. Viral Clearance Studies In accordance with Q5A, the rationale and action plan for assessing viral clearance and the results and evaluation of the viral clearance studies should be provided. Data can include those that demonstrate the validity of the scaled-down model compared to the commercial scale process; the adequacy of viral inactivation or removal procedures for manufacturing equipment and materials; and manufacturing steps that are capable of removing or inactivating viruses. (See related information in 3.2.S.2.5 and 3.2.P.3.5).

APPENDIX 4 TABLE OF CONTENTS FOR AN NDA IN USA

Besides the usual CTD sections which are requested for all ICH regions the following additional documents are requested for an NDA or BLA in USA[19]:

A. Module 1 - Administrative and Prescribing Information
Module 1 should contain all administrative documents (e.g., application forms, claims of categorical exclusion and certifications), and labeling, including the documents described below, as needed (Applicants often choose to submit a cover letter with their submissions. If you plan to include a cover letter, it should be placed at the beginning of Module 1.)
Documents should be organized in the order listed below. Generally, all of the documents in Module 1 can be provided in a single volume. Environmental assessments should be submitted separately.

1. FDA form 356h
The first document in Module 1 should be FDA form 356h.

2. Comprehensive table of contents
The next document in Module 1 should be the comprehensive table of contents for the entire submission. Each NDA and ANDA submission is required to have a comprehensive table of contents or index for the entire submission as described in 21 CFR 314.50 and 314.94. The comprehensive table of contents significantly enhances the usefulness of the document. It should include a complete list of all documents provided in the submission by module.
In the table of contents, you should identify the location of each document by referring to the volume numbers that contain the relevant documents and any tab identifiers. In general, the name for the tab identifier should be the name of the document (e.g., patent certification, financial disclosure) or section heading according to the CTD format (e.g., 3.2.P.4.2). If the full name of the document is too long for the tab identifiers, you should substitute an alternative name that adequately identifies the document. You should not use page numbers in the table of contents to refer to documents, but use tab identifiers as described above.

3. Administrative documents
a. Administrative documents
You should provide the appropriate administrative documents with the submission. Examples of administrative documents are listed below. See 21 CFR 314.50, 314.94, and 601.2 for details on the administrative documents

needed for specific submissions. FDA form 356h lists most of the administrative documents to be included in Module 1. The order of such documents should be consistent with that in FDA Form 356h.

- Patent information on any patent that claims the drug, if applicable
- Patent certifications (not for BLA)
- Debarment certification
- Field copy certification (not for BLA)
- User fee cover sheet
- Financial disclosure information

Letters of authorization for reference to other applications or drug master files

- Waiver requests
- Environmental assessment or request for categorical exclusion
- Statements of claimed exclusivity and associated certifications

Since these documents are small, you should place them in the same volume, separated by tab identifiers. If you submit an environmental assessment, you should provide it as a separate volume.

b. Prescribing information

You should include all copies of the labels and all labeling for the product in Module 1. The type of labeling provided depends on the submission. Examples of prescribing information include container and package labels as well as package inserts, draft labeling, patient leaflets, information sheets, and required Medication Guides. You should separate each sample of labeling by tab identifiers.

c. Annotated labeling text

For the NDA, you should provide a copy of the proposed labeling text with annotations directing reviewers to the information in the summaries and other modules that support each statement in the labeling, as described in 21 CFR 314.50(c)(2)(i). The annotated labeling text should include the content of the labeling described under 21 CFR 201.57 and all text, tables, and figures used in the package insert.

d. Labeling comparison

For the ANDA, you should provide the comparison of labeling that is described in 21 CFR 314.94(a)(8).

B. Module 2 – Common Technical Document Summaries

Module 2 should include the summary documents. You should provide the documents for this module in the order described below.

1. Overall CTD table of contents

For the first document in this module, you should provide a comprehensive table of contents listing all of the documents provided in the submission for modules 2 through 5.

2. Introduction to the summary documents

You should provide the introduction to the summary described in the guidance document M4: Organization of the CTD as a one page document.

3. Overviews and summaries

Module 2 should contain the following additional documents as described in the appropriate guidance documents (M4Q: The CTD -Quality, M4S: The CTD - Safety,

M4E: The CTD – Efficacy):

- Quality overall summary (2.3, Module 2, section 3)
- Non clinical overview (2.4)
- Clinical overview (2.5)
- Nonclinical summary (2.6)
- Clinical summary (2.7)

The nonclinical summary and the clinical summary should be provided in separate

volumes for ease of use by reviewers.

C. Module 3 - Quality

Module 3 should include information on the drug or biological substance and product that should be provided in the order described below. See Appendix A for additional recommendations on the content and organization of module 3.

1. Module 3 table of contents

The first document in this module should be a table of contents listing all of the documents provided for module 3. See the guidance document M4Q: The CTD Quality for the headings and order to be used in the table of contents, including numbering of section headings.

2. Body of data

Each individual subsection related to the drug or biological substance and product should be provided as an individual document either bound separately or divided by tab identifiers, depending on the size of the subsection. The *documents should be presented in the order in which they are listed in the table of contents.*

3. Literature References

Each literature reference should be provided as an individual document, separated from the others by tab identifiers.

D. Module 4 - Nonclinical Study Reports

Module 4 should contain the nonclinical study reports and related information. You should provide the documents for this module in the order described below.

1. Module 4 table of contents

The first document in this module should be a table of contents listing all of the documents provided for module 4. See the guidance to industry M4S: The CTD – Safety for the headings and order to be used in the table of contents, including numbering of section headings.

2. Study reports and related information

You should provide each study report and each related document as an individual document, separated from the other documents by binders or tab identifiers. These documents should be presented in the order in which they are listed in the table of contents.

3. Literature References

Each literature reference should be provided as an individual document, separated from the others by tab dividers.

<u>*E. Module 5 - Clinical Study Reports*</u>

Module 5 should contain clinical study reports and related information. You should provide the documents for this module in the order described below.

1. Module 5 table of contents

The first document in this module should be a table of contents listing all of the documents provided in Module 5. See the guidance to industry M4E: The CTD – Efficacy for the headings and order to be used in the table of contents, including numbering of section headings.

2. Study reports and related information

You should provide each study report and each related document, such as tabular listings of all clinical studies, as an individual document separated from the other documents by binders or tab dividers. We recommend that tab identifiers be provided for each appendix in a study report. These documents should be presented in the order in which they are listed in the table of contents.

The submission of a separate Integrated Summary of Efficacy (ISE) and/or Integrated Summary of Safety (ISS) is not required when the information provided can be incorporated into the CTD summaries and overview. When the ISS or ISE is submitted, it should be included in Module 5.3.5.3, Meta-Analyses. The applicant should raise any questions concerning the ISS and ISE with FDA staff prior to submission of the application.

You should include any case report forms (CRF) as separate documents. The case report forms should be organized by study.

The individual patient listings or case report tabulations (CRT) should include all of the clinical data collected in each study, organized by domain of data (e.g., adverse event, laboratory, physical examination). Each domain of data should be provided as a separate document. As with the CRFs, the CRTs should be organized by study.

3. Literature References

Each literature reference should be provided as an individual document separated from the others by tab identifiers.

APPENDIX 5 TABLE OF COMPARISON OF MECHANISMS TO HASTEN PRODUCT AVAILABILITY IN USA

Comparison of Mechanisms to Hasten Product Availability[22]:

	Accelerated review	Priority review	Fast track
Authority	1992 *Rule*: 21 CFR 314 and 601 (In 1997, Federal Food, Drug, and Cosmetic Act (FFDCA) 506(b).)	1996 Agency *Procedure*: CDER Manual of Policies and Procedures (MAPP) 6020.3; and CBER Manual of Standard Operating Procedures and Policies (SOPP) 8405	1997 *Statute*: FFDCA 506(a).
Procedure	[Not specified; presumably manufacturer would request and FDA would determine whether to grant.]	Clinical team leader of FDA review team, upon receipt of application, makes recommendation.	Any time before marketing approval, manufacturer requests designation; FDA grants if criteria are met.
Quality criteria	Serious or life-threatening illness	not applicable (n.a.)	Serious or life-threatening condition
	Potential to address unmet medical need	Major advance in treatment or treatment where no adequate therapy exists	Potential to address unmet medical need
	Adequate and well-controlled studies supporting use of surrogate outcome	n.a.	
Benefit during development	Adjusted trial outcome requirements	n.a.	Close communication with FDA
Benefit during review	n.a.	Additional attention; expedited review	Rolling review
Post approval requirements	Studies to extend results from surrogate to clinical outcome.	n.a.	

APPENDIX 6 TABLE OF SPECIFIC NATIONAL REQUIREMENTS OF NCADREAC DRAS CONCERNED

Country	Scope of the procedure	Timing of submission	Expected handling net time	Language of dossier	No. of copies to be submitted	Electronic submission	Need of samples and/or substances	Fees	Date of implementation
Bulgaria	Points 3.1, 3.2, and 3.3 of principles	Variant I	6 months, after receiving the complete documentation	English Bulgarian	1 copy 4 copies of SPC (in Bulgarian language) 4 copies of PIL (in Bulgarian language) 4 copies of labeling (in Bulgarian language)	CD-ROM, together with paper documentation of identical content; After approval SPC and PIL (final approved version) in the Bulgarian language on a 3.5-inch floppy diskette using Word° for Windows	2 samples of the medicinal product presented in the outer packaging. reference substance (if referred to in the testing procedure)	MA (original medicinal product): *Bulgarian Drug Agency (BDA)* fee: 2532 BGN levs *Ministry of Health (MoH)* fee: 3 800 BGN levs MA (original medicinal product — for II, III, IV etc pharmaceutical form): BDA fee: 1884 BGN levs MoH fee: 950 BGN levs	date of publishing

Country	Scope of the procedure	Timing of submission	Expected handling net time	Language of dossier	No. of copies to be submitted	Electronic submission	Need of samples and/or sub-stances	Fees	Date of implementation
Bulgaria								MA (original medicinal product – for different quantity of active substance (strength)): BDA fee 1256 BGN levs MoH fee 420 BGN levs MA (generic medicinal product, included in Pharmacopoeia) Bulgarian Drug Agency (BDA) fee 1909 BGN leva Ministry of Health (MoH) fee 1700 BGN leva	

Country	Scope of the procedure	Timing of submission	Expected handling net time	Language of dossier	No. of copies to be submitted	Electronic submission	Need of samples and/or sub-stances	Fees	Date of implementation
Bulgaria								MA (generic medicinal product included in Pharmacopoeia – for II, III, IV etc pharmaceutical form): *BDA fee*: 1432 BGN leva *MoH fee*: 425 BGN leva MA (generic medicinal product included in Pharmacopoeia – for different quantity of active substance (strength)): *BDA fee*: 955 BGN leva *MoH fee*: 420 BGN leva MA (generic medicinal product non-included in Pharmacopoeia):	

Country	Scope of the procedure	Timing of submission	Expected handling net time	Language of dossier	No. of copies to be submitted	Electronic submission	Need of samples and/or sub-stances	Fees	Date of implementation
Bulgaria								Bulgarian Drug Agency (BDA) fee: 2110 BGN leva Ministry of Health (MoH) fee: 1700 BGN leva MA (generic medicinal product non-included in Pharmaco-poeia – for II, III, IV, etc pharmaceutical form): BDA fee: 1583 BGN leva MoH fee: 425 BGN leva	

Country	Scope of the procedure	Timing of submission	Expected handling net time	Language of dossier	No. of copies to be submitted	Electronic submission	Need of samples and/or sub-stances	Fees	Date of implementation
Bulgaria								MA (generic medicinal product non-included in Pharmaco-poeia – for different quantity of active substance (strength)). *BDA fee*: 1055 BGN leva *MoH fee*: 420 BGN leva VARs (in Bulgaria VARs are not divided to type IA and type IB yet): - type I: *BDA fee*: 75 BGN levs *MoH fee*: 100 BGN levs (there are exceptions from MoH fee)	

Country	Scope of the procedure	Timing of submission	Expected handling net time	Language of dossier	No. of copies to be submitted	Electronic submission	Need of samples and/or sub-stances	Fees	Date of implementation
Bulgaria								-type II. *BDA fee:* 202 BGN levs *MoH fee:* 100 BGN levs (in case of new indication *MoH fee:* 300 BGN levs) **REN procedure:** original medicinal product *Bulgarian Drug Agency (BDA) fee:* 1266 BGN levs *Ministry of Health (MoH) fee:* 3040 BGN levs	

Country	Scope of the procedure	Timing of submission	Expected handling net time	Language of dossier	No. of copies to be submitted	Electronic submission	Need of samples and/or sub-stances	Fees	Date of implementation
Bulgaria								original medicinal product – for II, III, IV etc pharmaceutical for): *BDA fee*: 942 BGN levs *MoH fee*: 760 BGN levs ¶ original medicinal product – for different quantity of active substance (strength): *BDA fee*: 628 BGN levs ¶ *MoH fee*: 336 BGN levs	

190

Country	Scope of the procedure	Timing of submission	Expected handling net time	Language of dossier	No. of copies to be submitted	Electronic submission	Need of samples and/or sub-stances	Fees	Date of implementation
Bulgaria								generic medicinal product included in Pharmacopoeia: *Bulgarian Drug Agency (BDA) fee: 954.5 BGN levs* *Ministry of Health (MoH) fee: 1360 BGN levs* MA (generic medicinal product included in Pharmacopoeia – for II, III, IV etc pharmaceutical form): *BDA fee: 716 BGN levs* *MoH fee: 340 BGN levs*	

Country	Scope of the procedure	Timing of submission	Expected handling net time	Language of dossier	No. of copies to be submitted	Electronic submission	Need of samples and/or substances	Fees	Date of implementation
Bulgaria								generic medicinal product included in Pharmaco-poeia — for different quantity of active substance (strength). BDA fee 477.5 BGN levs MoH fee 336 BGN levs generic medicinal product non-included in Pharmaco-poeia Bulgarian Drug Agency (BDA) fee 1055 BGN levs Ministry of Health (MoH) fee 1360 BGN levs	

Country	Scope of the procedure	Timing of submission	Expected handling net time	Language of dossier	No. of copies to be submitted	Electronic submission	Need of samples and/or substances	Fees	Date of implementation
Bulgaria								generic medicinal product non-included in Pharmaco-poeia – for II, III, IV etc pharmaceutical form ¶ *BDA fee*: 769 BGN levs ¶ *MoH fee*: 340 BGN levs ¶ ¶ generic medicinal product non-included in Pharmaco-poeia – for different quantity of active substance (strength) ¶ *BDA fee*: 527.5 BGN levs ¶ *MoH fee*: 336 BGN levs	

Country	Scope of the procedure	Timing of submission	Expected handling net time	Language of dossier	No. of copies to be submitted	Electronic submission	Need of samples and/or sub-stances	Fees	Date of implementation
Bulgaria								THERE ARE FIXED EXCHANGE RATES OF Euro against the Bulgarian Lev (1 Euro is appr. 1.95583 LEV (BGNN))	
Croatia	Point 3.1	Variant	6 months, after receiving the complete documentation	English, Croatian	1 copy	Modules 1-3 in paper, modules 4 and 5 on CD-ROM, SPC, PIL and labeling in paper version	2 samples + reference substance	MA: 2 800 € VARs: type I: 240 €, type II 900€, Transfer of MA: 240 €	date of publishing

Country	Scope of the procedure	Timing of submission	Expected handling-net time	Language of dossier	No. of copies to be submitted	Electronic submission	Need of samples and/or sub-stances	Fees	Date of implementation
Romania	Points 3.1 and 3.3 of principles	Variant I	6 months, after receiving the complete documentation	English, Romanian	1 copy	possible submission of the dossier in Word, pdf, rtf, jpg and tiff format; CD-ROM, together with paper documentation of identical content, ¶ SPC and PIL (final approved version) in the Romanian language on a 3,5 inch floppy diskette using Word° for Windows	2 samples of the medicinal product presented in the outer packaging. ¶ reference substance (if referred to in the testing procedure)	MA: ¶ - new active substance ¶ - known ° active substance with BE studies 1420 € ¶ - known ° active substance without BE studies 1055 € ¶ - combination in fixed doses 1840 € ¶ - well established use (WEU) 1540 € ¶ VARs: ¶ - type IA: 210 € ¶ - type IB: 330 € ¶ - type II: 460 € ¶ Transfer of MA 300 €	

APPENDIX 7 INFORMATION SHARING LETTER

Text in italics should be replaced by the data specific to individual submissions.

Name of the product:
Mutual Recognition Procedure No.:

Approval of Information Sharing between the *DRA of the Reference Member State* and the *nCADREAC DRA*

The *Marketing Authorisation Holder (Drug Master File Holder) in the Reference Member State* hereby notifies to the *DRA of the Reference Member State* of the submission of an application for the marketing authorisation of the following medicinal product to the *nCADREAC DRA*:

name of the medicinal product, dosage form, strength, package size/s

(differences in brand name, if any)

proposed marketing authorisation holder in the country of the nCADREAC DRA

The *Marketing Authorisation Holder (Drug Master File Holder) in the Reference Member State* agrees that the *DRA of the Reference Member State* may make available to the *nCADREAC DRA* any information concerning the quality, safety and efficacy of the above product. The extent of this information shall not exceed that which is made available to EU Member States. In the case that variant II of this simplified procedure is used, the *Marketing Authorisation Holder (Drug Master File Holder) in the Reference Member State* agrees with the participation of the nCADREAC expert in the break out session.

The information will be used by the *nCADREAC DRA* in accordance with applicable laws and regulations for the marketing authorisation and safe use of medicinal products in the *country of the nCADREAC DRA*.

This Declaration is made as of the date first written below and remains valid for the period during which the product is authorised in the Member States of the EU and *the country of the nCADREAC DRA* respectively.

The copy of this declaration is sent to the nCADREAC DRA.

Date: Signature of the Marketing Authorisation Holder (Drug Master File Holder)
First name, family name:
Address:

APPENDIX 8 REPORT ON THE REPORT ON THE MARKETING AUTHORISATION GRANTED BY THE NCADREAC DRA CONCERNED OF THE MEDICINAL PRODUCT SUBJECTED TO THE MUTUAL RECOGNITION PROCEDURE IN THE EU

Text in italics should be replaced by the data specific to individual submissions.

nCADREAC DRA

TO: *DRA of the Reference Member State*

REPORT ON THE MARKETING AUTHORISATION GRANTED BY THE nCADREAC DRA CONCERNED OF THE MEDICINAL PRODUCT SUBJECTED TO THE MUTUAL RECOGNITION PROCEDURE IN THE EU

Name of the product in the RMS, pharmaceutical form/s, strength/s relevant to this report

INN or common name of the active ingredient/s

MRP number/s of the product

Name of the MA holder in the RMS

☐ Report on acceptance/REN of the MRP MA

☐ Report on disagreement with the MRP MA*

☐ Report on refusal of VAR*

☐ Report on retrospective inclusion of the product in the simplified nCADREAC system

☐ Request to RMS*

Name of the product in the nCADREAC DRA's country concerned

National Marketing authorisation number/s

Date of issue of national marketing authorisation decision

Name of the marketing authorisation holder in the nCADREAC DRA's country concerned

Authorised dosage forms, strengths, package sizes in nCADREAC DRA's country concerned

Modifications of SPC and PIL (specifying differences, except different name of the product, MA holder, national MA number)

Modifications of labelling (specifying differences, except different name of the product, MA holder, national MA number)

Explanatory notes*:

Enclosures:

Date   Signature of the person responsible within the nCADREAC DRA

APPENDIX 9   TABLE OF CONTENTS FOR ACTD

Part I: Table of Contents (ToC), Administrative Data and Product Information
The part I contains at the beginning an overall ToC of the whole ACTD which provided overall information of the dossier. After the ToC the administrative documents are contained. Administrative data can vary from country to country based on local requirements. Typical administrative data are application forms, CPPs, label, package inserts, etc. At the last section of part I the product information including prescribing information, pharmacological class, mode of action, adverse drug reactions,... is contained.
It is divided in the following sections:
- Section A: Introduction
- Section B: Overall ASEAN CTD ToC
- Section C: Documents required for registration (e.g. application forms, CPP, labeling, Product Data Sheet, prescribing information)

Part II: Quality Document
This part contains the QOS followed by the quality documents (DS and DP). The quality control documents should be described as much as possible.
It is divided in the following sections:
- Section A: ToCs
- Section B: QOS
- Section C: Body of Data

Part III: Nonclinical Document
This part begins with the nonclinical overview, followed by the nonclinical written summaries and the nonclinical tabulated summaries. The study reports may not be required for NCEs and biotechnological products if the original product is already authorized in the reference countries. An authority should ask for the necessary documents in case of a request for specific study reports.

It is divided in the following sections:
- Section A: ToCs
- Section B: NCO
- Section C: Nonclinical Written and Tabulated Summaries
  1. ToCs
  2. Pharmacology
  3. Pharmacokinetics
  4. Toxicology
- Section D: Nonclinical Stud Reports
  1. ToCs
  2. Pharmacology
  3. Pharmacokinetics
  4. Toxicology

Part IV: Clinical Document

This part contains the clinical overview and the clinical summary. The study reports may not be required for NCEs and biotechnological products if the original product is already authorized in the reference countries. An authority should ask for the necessary documents in case of a request for specific study reports.

It is divided in the following sections:
- Section A: ToCs
- Section B: CO
- Section C: Clinical Summary
  1. Summary of Biopharmaceutics and Associated Analytical Methods
  2. Summary of Clinical Pharmacology Studies
  3. Summary of Clinical Efficacy
  4. Summary of Clinical Safety
  5. Synopses of Individual Studies
- Section D: Tabular Listing of All Clinical Studies
- Section E: Clinical Study Reports
- Section F: List of Key Literature References

APPENDIX 10 DOSSIER REQUIREMENTS FOR QUALITY PART OF THE DOSSIER FOR ASEAN COUNTRIES

No.	Parameter	Components	Requirements	
			NCE	Biotech
S	**DRUG SUBSTANCE**			
S1	General information			
	1.1. Nomenclature	Information from S1	X	X
	1.2. Structure	1) Structural formula, including relative and absolute stereochemistry, the molecular formula, and the relative molecular mass	X	X
		2) Schematic amino acid sequence indicating glycosylation sites or other posttranslational modifications and relative molecular mass as appropriate		
	1.3. General Properties	Physico-chemical characteristics and other relevant properties including biological activity for biotech	X	X
S2	Manufacturer			
	2.1. Manufacturer(s)	Name and address of the manufacturer(s)	X	X
	2.2. Description of the manufacturing process and process control	1) The description of the drug substance manufacturing process and process control that represents the applicant's commitment for the manufacture of the drug substances.	X	X
				X
		2) Information on the manufacturing process, which typically starts with a vial(s) of the cell bank, and includes cell culture, harvest(s), purification and modification reaction, filling, storage and shipping conditions		
	2.3. Control of materials	1) Starting materials, solvents, reagents, catalysts, and any other materials used in the manufacture of the drug substance indicating where each material is used in the process. Tests and acceptance criteria of these materials.	X	X
				X
				X
			X	X

No.	Parameter	Components	Requirements	
		2) Control of source and starting materials of biological origin	X	
		3) Source, history and generation of cell substrate		
		4) Cell bank system, characterization and testing		
		5) Viral safety evaluation		
	2.4. Controls of critical steps and intermediates	1) Critical steps: Test and acceptance criteria with justification	X	X
		Including experimental data, performed at critical steps of the manufacturing process to ensure that the process is controlled	X	X X
		2) Intermediates: Specifications and analytical procedure, if any, for intermediates isolated during the process		
		3) Stability data supporting storage conditions		
	2.5. Process validation and/or evaluation	Process validation and/or evaluation studies for aseptic processing and sterilization	X	X
	2.6. Manufacturing process development	1) Description and discussion of significant changes made to the manufacturing process and/or manufacturing site of the drug substance used in producing non-clinical, clinical, scale-up, pilot and if available, production scale batches	X	X X
		2) The development history of the manufacturing process as described in S.2.2.		
S3	Characterization			
	3.1. Elucidation of structure and other characteristics	1) Confirmation of structure based on e.g. synthetic route and spectral analyses	X	X
		2) Details on primary, secondary and higher-order structure and information on biological activity, purity and immunochemical properties (when relevant)		

No.	Parameter	Components	Requirements	
	3.2. Impurities	Summary of impurities monitored or tested for during and after manufacture of drug substance	X	X
S4	Control of drug substance			
	4.1. Specifications	1) Detailed specification, tests and acceptance criteria	X	X
		2) Specify source, including as appropriate species of animal, type of microorganism, etc.		X
	4.2. Analytical procedures	The analytical procedures used for testing of drug substance	X	X
	4.3. Validation of analytical procedures	Analytical validation information, including experimental data for the analytical procedures used for testing of drug substance	X	X
	4.4. Batch analysis	Description of batches and results of the analysis to establish the specifications	X	X
	4.5. Justification of specification	Justification for drug substance specifications	X	X
S5	Reference standards or materials	Information on the reference standards or reference materials used for testing of the drug substance	X	X
S6	Container Closure System	Description of the container closure systems	X	X
S7	Stability	Stability report	X	X
P	**DRUG PRODUCT**			
P1	Description and Composition	1) Description	X	X
		2) Composition	X	X
		Name, quantity stated in metric weight or measures, function and quality standard reference		
P2	Pharmaceutical Development			
	2.1. Information on development studies	Data on the development studies conducted to establish that the dosage form, formulation, manufacturing process, container closure system, microbiological attributes and usage instruction are appropriate for the purpose specified in the application	X	X

No.	Parameter	Components	Requirements	
	2.2. Components of the drug product	Active ingredient		
		• Justification of the comparability of the active ingredient with excipients listed in P1	X	X
		• In case of combination products, justification of comparability of active ingredients with each other	X	X
		Excipients		
		• Justification for the choice of excipients listed in P1, which may influence the drug product performance		
	2.3. Finished product	Formulation Development	X	X
		• A brief summary describing the development of the finished product (taking into consideration the proposed route of administration and usage of NCE and Biotech)	X	X
		Overages		
		• Justification for any overage in the formulation(s) described in P1	X	X
		Physiochemical and biological properties		
		• Parameters relevant to the performance of the finished product, e.g. pH, dissolution		
	2.4. Manufacturing process development	1) Selection and optimization of the manufacturing process	X	X
			X	X
		2) Differences between the manufacturing process(es) used to produce pivotal clinical batches and the process described in P.3.2., if applicable		
	2.5 Container Closure System	Suitability of the container closure system used for the storage, transportation (shipping) and used for finished product	X	X
	2.6. Microbiological Attributes	Microbiological attributes of the dosage form, where appropriate	X	X

No.	Parameter	Components	Requirements	
	2.7. Compatibility	Compatibility of the finished product with reconstitution diluent(s) or dosage devices	X	X
P 3	Manufacture			
	3.1. Batch formula	Name and quantities of all ingredients	X	X
	3.2. Manufacturing process and process control	Description of manufacturing process and process control	X	X
	3.3. Control of critical steps and intermediates	Test and acceptance criteria	X	X
	3.4. Process validation and/or evaluation	Description, documentation and results of the validation and/or evaluation studies for critical steps or critical assays used in the manufacturing process	X	X
P4	Control of excipients			
	4.1. Specifications	Specifications for excipients	X	X
	4.2. Analytical procedures	Analytical procedures used for testing excipients where appropriate	X	X
	4.3. Excipient of human or animal origin	Information regarding sources and/or adventitious agents	X	X
	4.4. Novel excipients	For excipient(s) used the first time in a finished product or by a new route of administration, full details of manufacture, characterization and controls, with cross reference to supporting safety data (non-clinical or clinical)	X	X
P5	Control of drug product			
	5.1. Specifications	Specifications for the finished product	X	X
	5.2. Analytical procedures	Analytical procedures used for testing the finished product	X	X
	5.3. Validation of analytical procedures	Analytical validation information, including experimental data for the analytical procedures used for testing of the finished product	X	X
		Non compendial method	X	X
	5.4. Batch analysis	Description and test results of all relevant batches	X	X

No.	Parameter	Components	Requirements	
	5.5. Characterization of impurities	Information on characterization of impurities	X	X
	5.6. Justification of specification	Justification for the proposed finished product specification(s)	X	X
P6	Reference standard or materials	Information on the reference standards or reference materials used for testing of the finished product	X	X
P7	Container Closure System	Specification and control of primary and secondary packaging material, type of packaging and the package size, details of packaging inclusion (e.g. desiccant, etc.)	X	X
P8	Stability	Stability report: data demonstrating that product is stable through its proposed shelf life Commitment on post approval stability monitoring	X	X

APPENDIX 11 DOSSIER REQUIREMENTS FOR AN NCE IN CHINA

II Application Dossier Items
A Summary
1) Name of the drugs.
2) Certified Documents.
3) Objectives and basis for R & D.
4) Summary of main study work.
5) Draft of packaging insert, note to the draft, and latest literature.
6) Design of packaging and labeling.

B Pharmaceutical data
7) Summary of Pharmaceutical Study,
8) Research information and relevant literature of the production process of the drug substance, research information and relevant literature of formula and process of the preparations.
9) Study information and relevant literature for the chemical structure and components determination.
10) Study information and literature for quality specification.
11) Draft of quality specification and notes, and providing reference standard.
12) Test report of drug sample.
13) The source, test report and quality specification of drug substance and excipient.
14) Stability study and relevant literature.
15) Selection basis and quality specification of immediate packing material and container.

C Pharmacology and toxicology study information.
16) Summary of pharmacology and toxicology study.
17) Primary pharmacodynamics study and literature.
18) General Pharmacology study and literature.
19) Acute/single dose toxicity study and literature.
20) Repeated dose toxicity study and literature.
21) Special safety study and literature of hypersensitive (topical, systemic and photo-toxicity), hemolytic and topical irritative (blood vessel, skin, mucous membrane, and muscle) reaction related to topical and systemic use of the drugs.

22) Study and relevant literature on Pharmacodynamics, toxicity and pharmacokinetics change caused by the interactions amongst multiple components in the combination products.

23) Study and literature of mutagenicity test.

24) Study and literature of reproductive toxicity.

25) Study and literature of carcinogenicity test.

26) Study and literature of drug dependence.

27) Study and literature of pre-clinical pharmacokinetics.

D Clinical Study Information

28) Summary of global clinical study information.

29) Clinical study protocol.

30) Investigator's Brochure.

31) Draft of Informed Consent Form, approval of the Ethics Committee.

32) Clinical study report.

APPENDIX 12 TABLE OF APPLICATION INFORMATION ITEM FOR CHINA

Information category	information item	Registration category and information item requirement					
		1	2	3	4	5	6
Summary information	1	+	+	+	+	+	+
	2	+	+	+	+	+	+
	3	+	+	+	+	+	+
	4	+	+	+	+	+	+
	5	+	+	+	+	+	+
	6	+	+	+	+	+	+
Pharmaceutical Information	7	+	+	+	+	+	+
	8	+	*4	+	+	*4	*4
	9	+	+	+	+	+	+
	10	+	+	+	+	+	+
	11	+	+	+	+	+	+
	12	+	+	+	+	+	+
	13	+	+	+	+	+	+
	14	+	+	+	+	+	+
	15	+	+	+	+	+	+
		1	2	3	4	5	6
Pharmacology and toxicology	16	+	+	+	+	+	+
	17	+	*14	±	*16	—	—
	18	+	*14	±	*16	—	—
	19	+	*14	±	*16	—	—
	20	+	*14	±	*16	—	—
	21	*17	*17	*17	*17	*17	*17
	22	*11	—	—	—	—	—
	23	+	±	±	±	—	—
	24	+	±	±	±	—	—
	25	*6	—	*6	*6	—	—
	26	*7	—	—	—	—	—
	27	+	*18	*18	+	*18	—
Study informat	28	+	+	+	+	+	+
	29	+	+	+	+	+	△

208

Information category	Information item	Registration category and information item requirement					
		1	2	3	4	5	6
	30	+	+	+	+	+	△
	31	+	+	+	+	+	△
	32	+	+	+	+	+	△

Notes:

1. *+ Denote the information must be submitted,*
2. *± Denote literature can be used instead of test information,*
3. *– Denote the information may be exempted,*
4. ** Denote the information shall be submitted according to the requirement, *6 refer to note 6.*
5. *△denote that the provisions 4 of "V, Requirement For Clinical Study" shall apply.*
6. *literature refers to literature and / or summary of literature of all Pharmacology and toxicology study information of the drug in the application (including pharmacodynamic, mechanism of action, general pharmacology and toxicology and pharmacokinetics)"*

APPENDIX 13 DOSSIER REQUIREMENTS FOR AN NBE IN CHINA

    A   *Summary information*
1) *Name of the drugs.*
2) *Certified Documents.*
3) *Objectives and basis for the application.*
4) *Summary and evaluation of main research results.*
5) *Sample draft of insert sheet, notes to the draft, and literature.*
6) *Sample design for packing, label.*

    B   *Pharmaceutical Study Information*
7) *Summary of Pharmaceutical Study Information.*
8) *Research information of the raw material used for production.*
   i) *Research information about the sourcing, collection, and quality control of the animal or plant tissues or cells, unprocessed blood plasma.*
   ii) *Research information about the sourcing, collection (or selection) process, and determining of cells used for production.*
   iii) *Information about the establishment, determination, and storage of the strains banks, as well as the stability of transfer of culture.*
   iv) *Research information about the sourcing, quality control of other raw materials used for production.*
9) *Research information about the production process of the raw materials or the unprocessed fluids.*
10) *Research information of the formula and process of the preparations, source and quality standards of the supplementives, as well as the relevant literatures.*
11) *Experiment information and literature of the quality study of the products, including the preparing and standardizing of the Standard Material or Controls, as well as the comparison information with those similar product already marketed at domestic or overseas.*
12) *Record of manufacturing and testing of the sample products to be used for application of clinical study.*
13) *Draft of the manufacture and test standards, with notes to the draft and verification information of the test method.*
14) *Preliminary research information about the stability.*
15) *Basis for selection and quality standards of immediate packing material and container.*

C   Pharmacology and Toxicology Study Information

16) Summary about the pharmacology and toxicology study information.
17) Experiments information and literature of pharmacodynamic.
18) Experiments information and literature of regular pharmacology study.
19) Experiments information and literature of acute toxicity.
20) Experiments information and literature of long term toxicity.
21) Experiments information and literature of animal pharmacokinetics.
22) Experimental data and literature of mutations test.
23) Experimental data and literature of reproductive toxicity.
24) Experimental data and literature of carcinogenicity test.
25) Research information and literature of immunotoxicity and / or immunogenicity.
26) Experiments information and literature on major special safety test information related to topical and systemic use of the drugs, such as hemolysis and topical (blood vessel, skin, mucous membrane, endometium, tunica and muscle) irritation.
27) Experiments information and literature of the efficacy, toxicity and pharmacokinetics caused by the interactions between multiple components in the combination products.
28) Experiment information and literature of drug dependence.

D   Clinical Study Information

29) Summary of clinical study at domestic and overseas.
30) Clinical study plan and protocol.
31) Investigator's Brochure.
32) Sample draft of Informed Consent Form, approval of the ethics committee.
33) Summary report of the clinical study.

E   Others

34) Brief summary of the pre-clinical study.

35) Experiments and study information and summary of the production process improvement, quality perfection, the pharmacology and toxicology study and other works conducted during the clinical study.

36) Amendments and basis to amend of the approved manufacturing and testing standards.

37) Research and study information of the stability test.

38) Manufacturing and testing records of the 3 consecutive batches of trial products.

APPENDIX 14 TABLE OF APPLICATION INFORMATION ITEMS FOR CHINA

A Table of Application Information Items for therapeutic biological products, (Information Items 1-15, 29-38)

Info Cat.	Info Item	Registration category and requirement for information													
		1	2	3	4	5	6	7	8	9	10	11	12	13	14	15
Summary Information	1	+	+			+	+	+	+	+	+	+	+	+	+	+
	2	+	+			+	+	+	+	+	+	+	+	+	+	+
	3	+	+			+	+	+	+	+	+	+	+	+	+	+
	4	+	+			+	+	+	+	+	+	+	+	+	+	+
	5	+	+			+	+	+	+	+	+	+	+	+	+	+
	6	+	+			+	+	+	+	+	+	+	+	+	+	+
pharmaceutical	7	+	+	Refer to Technical guidance	Refer to Technical guidance	+	+	+	+	+	+	+	—	+	—	+
	8	+	+			+	—	+	+	+	+	+	—	—	—	+
	9	+	+			+	—	+	+	+	+	+	—	—	—	+
	10	+	+			+	+	+	+	+	+	+	—	+	—	+
	11	+	+			+	+	+	+	+	+	+	—	+	—	+
	12	+	+			+	+	+	+	+	+	+	—	+	—	+
	13	+	+			+	+	+	+	+	+	+	—	+	—	+
	14	+	+			+	+	+	+	+	+	+	—	+	—	+
	15	+	+			+	+	+	+	+	+	+	—	+	—	+
CT Info	29	+	+			+	+	+	+	+	+	+	+	+	+	+
	30	+	+			+	+	+	+	+	+	+	+	+	+	+
	31	+	+			+	+	+	+	+	+	+	+	+	+	+
	32	+	+			+	+	+	+	+	+	+	+	+	+	+
	33	+	+			+	+	+	+	+	+	+	+	+	+	+
other	34	+	+			+	+	+	+	+	+	+	+	+	+	+
	35	+	+			+	+	+	+	+	+	+	+	+	+	+
	36	+	+			+	+	+	+	+	+	+	—	+	—	+
	37	+	+			+	+	+	+	+	+	+	—	+	—	+
	38	+	+			+	+	+	+	+	+	+	—	+	—	+

Notes: 1. + denote the information must be submitted,
2. — denote the information may be exempted,
3. ± denote the information required or not required based on the particular case.

B	Table of Application Information Items for pharmacology and toxicology information for therapeutic biological product (Information Items 14-29)

Cat.	Item	Registration category and requirement for information														
		1	2	3	4	5	6	7	8	9	10	11	12	13	14	15
Pharmacology & Toxicology	16	+	+	Refer to Technical guidance	Refer to Technical guidance	+	+	+	+	+	+	+	+	+	+	+
	17	+	+			+	+	+	+	+	+	+	+	+	+	+
	18	+	+			+	+	+	+	+	+	+	+	+	+	+
	19	+	+			+	+	+	+	+	+	+	+	+	+	±
	20	+	+			+	+	+	+	+	+	+	+	+	+	+
	21	+	+			±	±	±	—	+	±	+	+	±	+	±
	22	±	±			±	±	±	—	±	±	±	±	—	±	—
	23	±	±			±	±	±	—	±	±	±	±	—	±	—
	24	±	±			±	±	±	—	±	±	±	±	—	±	—
	25	+	+			+	+	+	—	+	+	+	+	—	+	±
	26	+	+			+	+	+	—	+	+	+	+	+	+	±
	27	—	—			—	+	—	—	—	—	—	—	—	—	—
	28	±	±			±	—	—	—	±	—	—	±	—	—	—

Notes:
1. + denote the information must be submitted,
2. — denote the information may be exempted,
3. ± denote the information required or not required based on the particular case."

Requirements regarding clinical studies:

Item	Phase	Sample Size
Import Chemical Drug	PK	8 - 12
	Phase III	≥ 100 patients
Biological Drug	Phase I	20 (testing group)
	Phase II	100 (testing group)
	Phase III	300 (testing group)

Common MNC Practice for biological oncology product:
- Very few company goes through Phase I to III entirely
- The estimation of local study cases No. is based on experiences, specific indications, and could be discussed with local authority.

Smart Strategy Analysis:

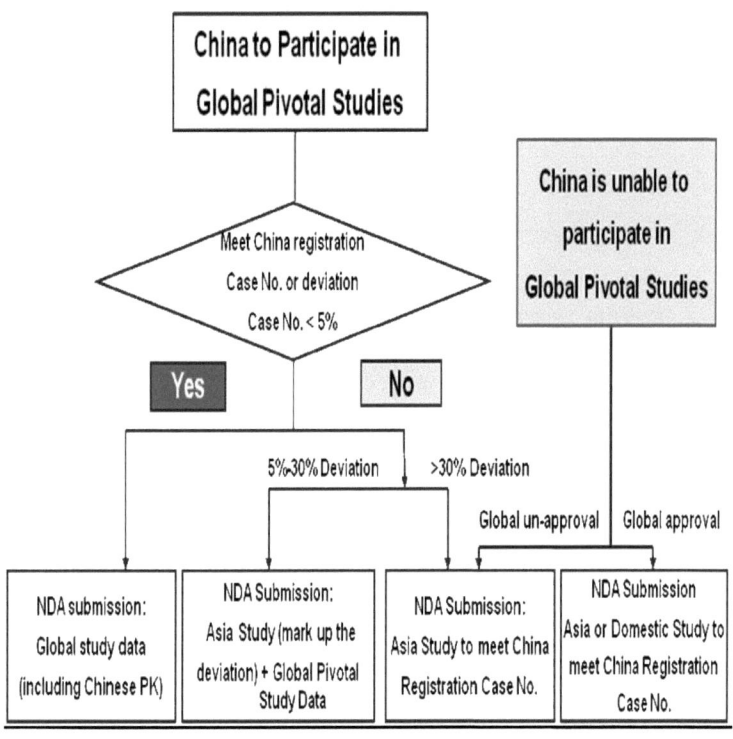

Strategy scenario analysis (high prevalence disease/indications):
➢ Best practice of registration case No. in China

Registration requirement	NCE		NBE
	New drug or new indication	New drug (not yet approved in China)	New indication (drug had been approved in China)
Case No. in pivotal study (testing group)	≥ 100 cases	≥ 200 cases	≥ 150 cases
Chinese PK data	≥ 8 - 12 cases	≥ 20 cases	≥ 20 cases

➢ Remark:
  o If the filing package contains more than one indication for NDA submission, the case No. in each indication can be decreased
  o PK data can be the PK profile from Phase III study

Strategy scenario analysis (rare or low incident disease/indications):

Situation	Regulatory Strategy
Orphan drug and rare diseases/indications	Clinical Trial Waiver application
Relatively low incident rate or late stage of diseases	Small scale local registration study or small cases No. in global study (local study: open, single arm, PK profile in certain No. of patients)

Key factors to achieve simultaneous regulatory approval:
➢ Integrate China into global regulatory plan (ideally after proof of concept)
➢ Involve China into global pivotal study and align appropriate Chinese patient number for registration
➢ Initiate Asia trial (bridging study) with main purpose for China registration and in parallel due to scientific issues (different epidemiology or etiology among different regions)
➢ Involve China medical & regulatory people at the early stage of drug development

APPENDIX 15 ADMINISTRATIVE DOCUMENTS ARE REQUIRED FOR NEW MEDICINAL PRODUCTS WHICH ARE IMPORTED TO BRAZIL

Requirement	New medicinal products (NCEs)	Biological products (NBEs)
Petition formularies	X	X
Receipt of payment of the respective fee or exemption document when applicable	X	X (additionally declaration of the size of the company)
Copy of the operative license	X	X (additionally copy of the operating authorization of the company
Copy of the register of the technical responsible professional at the professional council	X	X
Copy of the protocol of the notification of the pilot batches manufacturing dossier (for products manufactured in Brazil)	X	
Copy of operating authorization and of the special operating authorization, if applicable	X	
Information of the registration status of the product worldwide	X	X
CPP • Proof of the registration of the finished biological/chemical medicinal product in the manufacturing country or in another country • Proof of the commercialization of the product in the manufacturing country • Attachment the approved package insert	X	X
Letter of authorization (Power of Attorney)	X	X
GMP certificates: • issued by ANVISA or copy of the protocol of the inspection request for local manufacturer • issued by ANVISA for the production line of the manufacturer in Brazil (for products imported as bulk or in primary package into Brazil)	X	X

Requirement	New medicinal products (NCEs)	Biological products (NBEs)
• issued by the CAs in the country of manufacture (notarized copy is required) of bulk product, as product in the primary package or as finished biological/chemical medicinal product		
Manufacturing authorizations • for all manufacturing sites involved in the DS and DP manufacturing process	X	X
Authorization for the use of trademark	X	X
Information about the manufacturing stage of imported products: finished product, bulk or in primary packaging	X	X
Statement regarding the Batch code interpretation	X	X
Bar code for all marketing presentations		X
Document indicating: name and address of the manufacturers of: the biological active ingredient; the biological medicinal product in bulk; the biological medicinal product in the respective primary package; the finished biological medicinal product. Name and address of the manufacturer that issued the release certificate of the finished biological medicinal products batches		X
Copy of the documents that determines the product specifications for a finished biological medicinal product		X

APPENDIX 16 DOSSIER REQUIREMENTS (PHARMACEUTICAL/ CHEMICAL/ BIOLOGICAL, PRECLINICAL AND CLINICAL DOCUMENTATION) FOR BRAZIL

Requirements	New medicinal products (NCEs)	Biological products (NBEs)
Package insert (general information about the product including information about pharmaceutical form, formula, routes of administration, indications and contraindications, adverse reactions and others)	X	X
Mock-ups of the packaging materials	X	X
Production and quality control report containing information about the formula; summary of the manufacturing process; report on quality control with physicochemical, biological and microbiologic controls; analytical methods; information about the reference standards used and other detailed information:	X	X
• Amount of the components of the formula specified by their respective technical names Brazilian Common Denomination (DCB), DCI, INN or CAS, following the regulations in force	X X X X	X X X X
• Amount and role of each component in the formula expressed in the metric system or standard unit	X	X
• Inform the function of each component in the formula	X	X
• Maximum and minimum industrial batch size	X	X
• Description of the manufacturing process of the API and finished product and of the equipment used	X	X
• Description of the manufacturing process of the medicinal product in bulk	X	X
• In process control methods		X
• Criteria for batches identification		X
• Codification used by the manufacturer to identify the batches of the finished biological medicinal products		X
• Storage conditions and procedures used during transportation of the API; of the biological medicinal product in bulk; of the biological medicinal product in the primary package; of the finished biological medicinal product and respective storage conditions		X X X

Requirements	New medicinal products (NCEs)	Biological products (NBEs)
• Transport validation report of the product in the primary package and as finished biological medicinal product. • In case of thermolabil products add a declaration of the manufacturer that the transport complies with the cold chain requirements • Report on the viral inactivation process and the respective validation. For blood products. • Report on the sorology quality control process and reactive C protein, carried out with the plasma and respective validation. For blood products		
(*) Brazilian pharmacopoeia or other international codes accepted by the ANVISA (Resolution-RDC 79 of 11-Apr-2003 and Resolution RDC 169 of 21-Aug-2006		
API • Technical information: structure formula; molecular formula; molecular weight; synonymous; physical form; burning point; solubility; specific optical rotation; organoleptic properties; possible isomers; polymorphism; salt/base ratio; IR spectrum; other identification parameters used by the API manufacturer • Description of the manufacturing process of the API and of the equipment used • Detailed quality control report including physico- chemical, biological and microbiological analysis carried out with the API • Analytical methods and respective limits and reference standards used by the manufacturer • stability studies • list of solvents • list of residual solvents • respective concentrations	X	X
Manufacturing batch records of DP	X	X

Requirements	New medicinal products (NCEs)	Biological products (NBEs)
Quality control of raw materials • Detailed description of the specifications • Identification and quantification analytical methods of the formula components and of the major contaminants • For drops, the routine analytical tests and specifications for the device • Notes: reference values have to be described on official compendiums accepted by the ANVISA; in house methods have to be validated for the active ingredient. Translation is only required if the original language is not English or Spanish	X	X
Quality control of the finished product • Detailed analytical methods; specifications and respective bibliographic references; graphic representations of the dissolution profile, when applicable • Detailed quality control report including physico- chemical, biological and microbiological analysis carried out with the finished biological/chemical medicinal product • For imported biological medicinal products, analytical methods used by the importer	X X X	X X X
Certificates of analysis (CoAs) of DS and DP	X	X
Physical; chemical; biological and microbiological quality control methods to be carried out by the importer	X	X
Stability study • Description of the stability studies of the finished biological/chemical medicinal product to support the proposed expiry period • Stability studies should be carried out with at least 3 batches of the product in the same strength; pharmaceutical form; primary package and ambient conditions. • Studies results shall be presented in tables containing the physico-chemical; microbiological and chemical analysis; manufacturing date and batches codification identification	X	X

Requirements	New medicinal products (NCEs)	Biological products (NBEs)

• ANVISA accepts stability tests carried out based on the MCS and WHO criteria. EMA; ICH and FDA guidelines will be accepted as references.
• Accelerated stability study results of three batches and results of the ongoing long term studies
• Note: Accelerated: 40± 2°C/75 ±5%RH (storage temp.:15°C -30°C); Accelerated: 25±2°C/60±5% RH (storage temp.:2°C - 8°C)
• Please see Resolution RE 01/05 for detailed guidelines
• For medicinal products imported in bulks:
   o expiry period must take into consideration the maximum storage period until primary packaging
• For medicinal products imported in bulk or in the primary package:
   o follow up stability studies have to be carried out in Brazil		

BSE information • Resolution RDC 305/02 : accomplishment with the restrictions for products containing raw materials subject the current legislation referred to the BSE	X	X
Packaging materials specifications	X	X
Complementary information: • Inform the inscription of the substance or the basic formula components in formularies; pharmacopeias; standardizing official publications or any recognized scientific publication. • Bibliography • Advantages of the formula with the respective clinical rationale • Products in association of one or more substances have to add evidence of safety ,efficacy and benefits of the Association		X

Requirements	New medicinal products (NCEs)	Biological products (NBEs)
Pharmacodynamics • Mechanism of action • Dosage and administration • Rationale for the recommended dosage • Therapeutic index, when applicable	X	X
Pharmacokinetics (for each API of the formulation) • pKa • biological half-life • Absorption • Distribution • Biotransformation • Excretion/elimination	X	X
Pharmacovigilance data including Phase IV clinical studies results	X	X
Preclinical report • Acute and sub acute toxicity, chronic, reproductive toxicity, mutagenicity, oncogenic potential	X	X
Clinical studies: safety and efficacy • Phase I, II, III; Phase IV studies when applicable • Clinical studies being carried out in Brazil, have to include information about the status and who is responsible for. • The applicant may present clinical studies that demonstrate 'noninferiority" as a demonstration of the therapeutic indication and safety. • For new medicinal products associations and two or more marketing presentations in one package for concomitant or sequential use: rationale about the benefits of the combination and, when applicable, results of: comparative relative bioavailability among the API's in combination and each of the API's of the formula; clinical trials for each therapeutic indication to prove the additive or synergic effect of the combination	X X X X X X	X X X X

Requirements	New medicinal products (NCEs)	Biological products (NBEs)
with no increase of the risks involved. Depending on the case, when appropriate technical or ethical rationale is available, the clinical studies may be substituted or complemented by other alternative studies. • New therapeutic indication of a medicinal product already approved for marketing in Brazil for another company in the same strength and pharmaceutical form: Phase II clinical trials results • New strength; new pharmaceutical form; route of administration of a medicinal product already approved for marketing in Brazil for another company: Phases II and III. These studies may be replaced by relative bioavailability studies when in a therapeutic renage already approved for the product	X	
Price report • Provide price of the medicinal product in countries where it is marketed. In case the product is not marketed abroad, present price proposal • Note: Although there is no reimbursement in Brazil, the registration approval of a new medicinal product will not be granted without a price proposal of the applicant.	X	X

APPENDIX 17 ROUTE MAP FOR CREATION OF A CTD DOSSIER FOR MAA

CTD Structure MODULE 1	Author	First Draft [date]	Final Draft [date]	Submission ready-document [date]	M1 - Dossier-ID Dossier-ID Number	M1 Version No.	Comments	Lifecycle Attributes
1.4.2 Information about the expert - non clinical								
1.4.3 Clinical								
1.4.3 Information about the expert - clinical								
1.5 Specific requirements for different types of application								
1.5.1 Information for bibliographical applications								
1.5.2 Information for Generic, "Hybrid' or Bio-similar Applications								
1.5.3 (Extended) Data/market Exclusivity								
1.5.4 Exceptional Circumstances								
1.5.5 Conditional Marketing Authorisation								
1.6 Environmental Risk Assessment								
1.6 Environmental Risk Assessment								
1.6.1 Non-GMO								
1.6.2 GMO								
1.7 Information relating to Orphan Market Exclusivity								
1.7.1 Similarity								
1.7.2 Market Exclusivity								
1.8 Information relating to Pharmacovigilance								
1.8.1 Pharmacovigilance System								
1.8.2 Risk-management System								

CTD-Structure MODULE 1	Author	First-Draft [date]	Final-Draft [date]	Submission-ready-document [date]	M1-Dossier-Dossier-ID-Number	M1 Version No.	Comments	Lifecycle-Attributes
1.4.2 Information about the expert - non clinical								
1.4.3 Clinical								
1.4.3 Information about the expert - clinical								
1.5 Specific requirements for different types of application								
1.5.1 Information for bibliographical applications								
1.5.2 Information for Generic, "Hybrid" or Bio-similar Applications								
1.5.3 (Extended) Data/market Exclusivity								
1.5.4 Exceptional Circumstances								
1.5.5 Conditional Marketing Authorisation								
1.6 Environmental Risk Assessment								
1.6.1 Environmental Risk Assessment								
1.6.1 Non-GMO								
1.6.2 GMO								
1.7 Information relating to Orphan Market Exclusivity								
1.7.1 Similarity								
1.7.2 Market Exclusivity								
1.8 Information relating to Pharmacovigilance								
1.8.1 Pharmacovigilance System								
1.8.2 Risk-management System								

CTD Structure — MODULE 1

	Author	First Draft [date]	Final Draft [date]	Submission-ready-document [date]	M1 Dossier-DossierID-Number	M1 Version No.	Comments	Lifecycle Attributes
1.9 Information relating to Clinical Trials								
1.9 Information relating to Clinical Trials								
Additional data								
Manufacturing Authorisation of manufacturer								
QP Declaration of manufacturer								
Responses to Questions								

	Module 2							
2.1	CTD table of contents (Module 2-5)							
2.2	Introduction							
2.3	Quality Overall Summary							
2.3.1	Introduction							
2.3.S	Drug Substance							
2.3.P	Drug Product							
2.3.A	Appendices							
2.3.R	Regional Information							
2.4	Nonclinical overview							
2.4	Nonclinical overview							
2.5	Clinical overview							
2.5	Clinical Overview							
Annex 1	CIOMS Forms Arrest							
Annex 2	CIOMS line listing Arrest							
Annex 3	CIOMS Forms Infarction and Ischemia							
Annex 4	CIOMS line listing Infarction and Ischemia							
Annex 5	CIOMS Forms PE							
Annex 6	CIOMS line listing PE							
2.6	Nonclinical Summary							
2.6.1	Introduction							
2.6.2	Pharmacology Written Summary							
2.6.3	Pharmacology Tabulated Summary							
2.6.4	Pharmacokinetics Written Summary							
2.6.5	Pharmacokinetics Tabulated Summary							
2.6.6	Toxicology Written Summary							
2.6.7	Toxicology Tabulated Summary							
2.7	Clinical Summary							
2.7.1	Summary of Biopharmaceutic Studies and Associated Analytical Methods							
2.7.2	Summary of Clinical Pharmacology Studies							

Module 2										
2.7.3	Summary of Clinical Efficacy									
2.7.4	Summary of Clinical Safety									
2.7.5	Literature References									
2.7.6	Synopses of Individual Studies									

CTD-Structure MODULE 3		Author	First Draft [date]	Final Draft [date]	Submission-ready document [date]	M1-Dossier-Dossier-ID-Number	M1 Version-No.	Comments	Lifecycle-Attributes
3	Module 3 Quality								
3.1	Table of contents								
3.2	Body of data								
3.2.S	Drug Substance								
3.2.S.1	General information								
3.2.S.1.1	Nomenclature								
3.2.S.1.2	Structure								
3.2.S.1.3	General properties								
3.2.S.2	Manufacture								
3.2.S.2.1	Manufacturer(s)								
3.2.S.2.2	Description of manufacturing process and process controls								
3.2.S.2.3	Control of materials								
3.2.S.2.4	Controls of critical steps and intermediates								
3.2.S.2.5	Process validation and/or evaluation								
3.2.S.2.6	Manufacturing process development								
3.2.S.3	Characterization								
3.2.S.3.1	Elucidation of structure and other characteristics								
3.2.S.3.2	Impurities								
3.2.S.4	Control of drug substance								
3.2.S.4.1	Specification								
3.2.S.4.2	Analytical procedures								
3.2.S.4.3	Validation of analytical procedures								
3.2.S.4.4	Batch analyses								
3.2.S.4.5	Justification of specification								

CTD-Structure MODULE 3	Author	First Draft [date]	Final Draft [date]	Submission-ready document [date]	M1-Dossier-Dossier-ID-Number	M1 Version-No.	Comments	Lifecycle-Attributes
3.2.S.5	Reference standards or materials							
3.2.S.5	Reference standards or materials							
3.2.S.6	Container closure system							
3.2.S.6	Container closure system							
3.2.S.7	Stability							
3.2.S.7.1	Stability summary and conclusions							
3.2.S.7.2	Post-approval stability protocol and stability commitments							
3.2.S.7.3	Stability data							
3.2.P	Drug product							
3.2.P.1	Description and composition of the drug product							
3.2.P.2	Pharmaceutical development							
3.2.P.3	Manufacture							
3.2.P.3.1	Manufacturer(s)							
3.2.P.3.2	Batch formula							
3.2.P.3.3	Description of manufacturing process and process controls							
3.2.P.3.4	Control of critical steps (Description) and intermediates							
3.2.P.3.5	Process validation and/or evaluation							
3.2.P.4	Control of excipients							
3.2.P.4.1	Specifications							
3.2.P.4.2	Analytical procedures							
3.2.P.4.3	Validation of analytical procedures							
3.2.P.4.4	Justification of specification							

CTD Structure MODULE 3	Author	First Draft [date]	Final Draft [date]	Submission-ready document [date]	M1 Dossier-Dossier-ID-Number	M1 Version No.	Comments	Lifecycle Attributes
3.2.P.4.5	Excipients of human or animal origin							
3.2.P.4.6	Novel excipients							
3.2.P.5	Control of drug product							
3.2.P.5.1	Specification(s)							
3.2.P.5.2	Analytical procedures							
3.2.P.5.3	Validation of analytical procedures							
3.2.P.5.4	Batch analyses							
3.2.P.5.5	Characterization of impurities							
3.2.P.5.6	Justification of specification							
3.2.P.6	Reference standards or materials							
3.2.P.6	Reference standards or materials							
3.2.P.7	Container closure system							
3.2.P.7	Container closure system							
3.2.P.8	Drug product stability							
3.2.P.8.1	Stability summary and conclusion							
3.2.P.8.2	Post-approval stability protocol and stability commitments							
3.2.P.8.3	Stability data							
3.2.A	Appendices							
3.2.A.1	Facilities and equipment							
3.2.A.2	Adventitious safety evaluation							
3.2.A.3	Novel excipients							
3.2.R	Regional information							
3.2.R.1	Batch records							
3.2.R.2	Process validation scheme for Drug Product							
3.2.R.3	Medical Device							

CTD-Structure MODULE: 3	Author	First Draft [date]	Final-Draft [date]	Submission-ready document [date]	M1-Dossier-Dossier-ID-Number	M1 Version-No.	Comments	Lifecycle-Attributes
3.2.R.4	Materials of animal origin incl. Table A, B and C							
3	Literature references							
3.3.1.x								

CTD-Structure MODULE 4	Study Number	Author	First Draft [date]	Final Draft [date]	Submission-ready document [date]	M1-Dossier-Dossier-ID-Number	M1 Version-No.	Comments	Lifecycle-Attributes
4.	Module 4 Nonclinical study reports								
4.1	Table of contents								
4.2	Study reports								
4.2.1	Pharmacology								
4.2.1.1	Primary Pharmacodynamics								
4.2.1.1.x	Study reports								
4.2.1.2	Secondary Pharmacodynamics								
4.2.1.2.x	Study reports								
4.2.1.3	Safety Pharmacology								
4.2.1.3.x	Study reports								
4.2.1.4	Pharmacodynamic Drug Interactions								
4.2.1.4.x	Study reports								
4.2.2	Pharmacokinetics								
4.2.2.1	Analytical methods and validations reports								
4.2.2.1.x	Study reports								
4.2.2.2	Absorption								
4.2.2.2.x	Study reports								
4.2.2.3	Distribution								
4.2.2.3.x	Study reports								
4.2.2.4	Metabolism								
4.2.2.4.x	Study reports								
4.2.2.5	Excretion								
4.2.2.5.x	Study reports								
4.2.2.6	Pharmacokinetic drug interactions								
4.2.2.6.x	Study reports								
4.2.2.7	Other pharmacokinetic studies								
4.2.2.7.x	Study reports								

CTD-Structure MODULE 4	Study Number	Author	First Draft [date]	Final Draft [date]	Submission-ready document [date]	M1-Dossier Dossier-ID-Number	M1 Version No.	Comments	Lifecycle-Attributes
4.2.3	Toxicology								
4.2.3.1	Single-dose toxicity								
4.2.3.1.x	Study reports								
4.2.3.2	Repeated-dose toxicity								
4.2.3.2.x	Study reports								
4.2.3.3	In vitro								
4.2.3.3.1.x	Study reports								
4.2.3.3	In vivo								
4.2.3.3.2.x	Study reports								
4.2.3.4	Carcinogenicity								
4.2.3.4.x	Study reports								
4.2.3.4.1	Long-term studies								
4.2.3.4.1.x	Study reports								
4.2.3.4.2	Short- or medium-term studies								
4.2.3.4.2.x	Study reports								
4.2.3.4.3	Other studies								
4.2.3.4.3.x	Study reports								
4.2.3.5	Reproductive and developmental toxicity								
4.2.3.5.1	Fertility and early embryonic development								
4.2.3.5.1.x	Study reports								
4.2.3.5.2	Embryo-fetal development								
4.2.3.5.2.x	Study reports								
4.2.3.5.3	Prenatal and postnatal development								
4.2.3.5.3.x	Study reports								
4.2.3.5.3	Studies in which the offspring (juvenile animals) are dosed and/or further evaluated								
4.2.3.5.4.x	Study reports								
4.2.3.6	Local tolerance								
4.2.3.6.x	Study reports								

CTD-Structure MODULE 4	Study Number	Author	First Draft [date]	Final Draft [date]	Submission-ready document [date]	M1-Dossier Dossier-ID Number	M1 Version No.	Comments	Lifecycle Attributes
4.2.3.7 Other toxicity studies (if available)									
4.2.3.7.1 Antigenicity									
4.2.3.7.1.x Study reports									
4.2.3.7.2 Immunotoxicity									
4.2.3.7.2.x Study reports									
4.2.3.7.3 Mechanistic studies									
4.2.3.7.3.x Study reports									
4.2.3.7.4 Dependence									
4.2.3.7.4.x Study reports									
4.2.3.7.5 Metabolites									
4.2.3.7.5.x Study reports									
4.2.3.7.6 Impurities									
4.2.3.7.6.x Study reports									
4.2.3.7.7 Other									
4.2.3.7.7.x Study reports									
4.3 Literature references									
4.3.x									

CTD-Structure MODULE 5	Study Number	Authors	First Draft [date]	Final Draft [date]	Submission-ready document [date]	M1-Dossier-Dossier ID-Number	M1-Version No.	Comments	Lifecycle-Attributes
5									
5.1									
	Clinical Study Reports								
	Table of contents for clinical study reports								
5.2	Tabular Listing of all Clinical Studies								
5.3	Clinical study reports								
5.3.1	Reports of biopharmaceutic studies								
5.3.1.1	Bioavailability study reports								
5.3.1.1.x	Study reports								
5.3.1.2	Comparative bioavailability and bioequivalence study reports								
5.3.1.2.x	Study reports								
5.3.1.3	In vitro-in vivo correlation study reports								
5.3.1.3.x	Study reports								
5.3.1.4	Reports of Bioanalytical and Analytical Methods								
5.3.1.4.x	Study reports								
5.3.2	Reports of Studies Pertinent to Pharmacokinetics using Human Biomaterials								
5.3.2.1	Plasma Protein Binding Study Reports								
5.3.2.1.x	Study reports								
5.3.2.2	Reports of Hepatic Metabolism and Drug Interaction Studies								
5.3.2.2.x	Study reports								
5.3.2.3	Reports of Studies Using Other Human Biomaterials								
5.3.2.3.x	Study reports								
5.3.3	Reports of Human Pharmacokinetic (PK) Studies								

CTD Structure MODULE 5	Study Number	Author	First Draft [date]	Final Draft [date]	Submission-ready document [date]	M1-Dossier Dossier-ID Number	M1 Version No.	Comments	Lifecycle Attributes
5.3.3.x	Study reports								
5.3.3.1	Healthy Subject PK and Initial Tolerability Study Reports								
5.3.3.1.x	Study reports								
5.3.3.2	Patient PK and Initial Tolerability Study Reports								
5.3.3.2.x	Study reports								
5.3.3.3	Intrinsic Factor PK Study Reports								
5.3.3.3.x	Study reports								
5.3.3.4	Extrinsic Factor PK Study Reports								
5.3.3.4.x	Study reports								
5.3.3.5	Population PK Study Reports								
5.3.3.5.x	Study reports								
5.3.4	Reports of Human Pharmacodynamic (PD) Studies								
5.3.4.x	Study reports								
5.3.4.1	Healthy Subject PD and PK/PD Study Reports								
5.3.4.1.x	Study reports								
5.3.4.2	Patient PD and PK/PD Study Reports								
5.3.4.2.x	Study reports								
5.3.5	Reports of Efficacy and Safety Studies								
5.3.5.1	Study Reports of Controlled Clinical Studies Pertinent to the Claimed Indication								
5.3.5.1.x	Study reports								
5.3.5.2	Study Reports of Uncontrolled Clinical Studies								
5.3.5.2.x	Study reports								
5.3.5.3	Reports of Analyses of Data from More Than One Study								
5.3.5.3.x	Study reports								

CTD-Structure MODULE-5	Study Number	Author	First Draft [date]	Final Draft [date]	Submission-ready document [date]	M1-Dossier-Dossier-ID-Number	M1-Version No.	Comments	Lifecycle-Attributes
5.3.5.4	Other Study Reports								
5.3.5.4.x	Study reports								
5.3.6	Reports of Postmarketing Experience - not applicable								
5.3.6.x	Periodic Safety Update Reports								
5.3.7	Case Report Forms and Individual Patient Listings, When Submitted								
5.3.7.x	Study reports								
5.4	Literature references								
5.4.x									

APPENDIX 18 AN EXAMPLE FOR A GLOBAL PLAN:

Target: Monoclonal antibody which is EGFR targeting
INN: Monotuximab
Indications under development and stage of development:
Hodgkin lymphoma: Phase III clinical trial is ongoing
Squamous cancer of the head and neck (SCCHN): Phase II clinical trials ongoing
Breast cancer: Phase I clinical trials are ongoing

Example for a ToC:
Table of Content
List of Abbreviations
Executive Summary
Major changes since last global plan version (only applicable for updates of a global plan)
1 Decision(s) required
2 Product Vision
2.1 Compound Description
2.2 Vision
3 Product Objectives
3.1 Target Product Profile or Target Product Claims
3.2 Short, medium & long term objectives
4 Analysis of the situation
4.1 Data Summary (aspects common to all indications under development)
4.1.1 Brief Assessment of Intellectual Property Situation
4.1.2 Contractual Obligations with External Partners (only if applicable)
4.1.3 Manufacturing and supply summary
4.1.4 Non clinical summary
4.1.5 Regulatory summary
4.1.6 SWOT analysis
4.2 Data Summary (indication-specific aspects)
4.2.1 Hodgkin lymphoma
Clinical summary
Summary of competitive situation
4.2.2 Squamous cancer of the head and neck (SCCHN)
Clinical summary
Summary of competitive situation

4.2.3 Breast cancer

Clinical summary

Summary of competitive situation

5 Development Options considered for the current investment decision

5.1 Summary of Options considered

5.2. Hodgkin lymphoma

5.2.1 Summary/rationale of this option

5.2.2 Decision Tree and go/no go Criteria

5.2.3 Timelines, Resources, Costs and Sales

5.2.4 Evaluation of the options

5.3. SCCHN

5.3.1 Summary/rationale of SCCHN

5.3.2 Decision Tree and go/no go Criteria

5.3.3 Timelines, Resources, Costs and Sales

5.3.4 Evaluation of the options

Critical Success Factors

5.4. Breast cancer

5.4.1 Summary/rationale of this option

5.4.2 Decision Tree and go/no go Criteria

5.4.3 Timelines, Resources, Costs and Sales

5.4.4 Evaluation of the options

5.5. Indication IV (combination therapy) (only if applicable)

6 Details of/Strategy for recommended/endorsed option(s)

6.1 Recommendation

6.2 Rationale for Option SCCHN (Hodgkin lymphoma and/or Breast Cancer)

6.3 Scope of Work for Hodgkin lymphoma

6.3.1 Non clinical development strategy

6.3.2 Clinical development strategy

6.3.3 Regulatory development strategy

6.3.4 Commercial development strategy

6.3.5 Manufacturing and supply strategy

6.3.6 Key milestones

6.3.7 Critical Path Aspects

6.3.8 Criteria for passing next development point

6.4 Scope of Work for SCCHN

6.4.1 Non clinical development strategy

6.4.2 Clinical development strategy

6.4.3	Regulatory development strategy	
6.4.4	Commercial development strategy	
6.4.5	Manufacturing and supply strategy	
6.4.6	Key milestones	
6.4.7	Critical Path Aspects	
6.4.8	Criteria for passing next development point	
6.5	Scope of Work for Breast cancer	
6.5.1	Non clinical development strategy	
6.5.2	Clinical development strategy	
6.5.3	Regulatory development strategy	
6.5.4	Commercial development strategy	
6.5.5	Manufacturing and supply strategy	
6.5.6	Key milestones	
6.5.7	Critical Path Aspects	
6.5.8	Criteria for passing next development point	
7	Key Risks and Opportunities	
7.1	Threats & Opportunities – Probability and impact	
7.2	Action plans to minimize risks/maximize key opportunities	
8	Financial Analysis	
8.1	Key Assumptions and Sales Forecast	
8.2	Research and Development resources and costs	
8.3	Sales and Marketing resources and costs	
8.4	Cost of Goods	
8.5	Net present value & expected net present value	
9	Communication plan	
10	List of supporting documents	

APPENDIX 19 AVAILABLE GUIDELINES AND REGULATIONS

Quality guidelines

ICH documents

- ICH M4 Quality:
  Quality overall Summary and CTD Quality Rev 1
- ICH Q 1 A (R2):
  Stability Testing of New Drug Substances and Products
- ICH Q 1 B:
  Photostability Testing of New Active Substances and Medicinal products
- ICH Q 1 E:
  Evaluation of Stability Data
- ICH Q 2 A:
  Validation of Analytical Methods: Definitions and Terminology
- ICH Q 2 B:
  Validation of Analytical Procedures: Methodology
- ICH Q 3 A (R):
  Impurities Testing: Impurities in New Drug Substances
- ICH Q 3 B (R):
  Impurities in New Medicinal Products
- ICH Q 3 C:
  Impurities: Residual Solvents
- ICH Q 6 A:
  Specifications: Test procedures and Acceptance Criteria for New Drug Substances and New Drug Products: Chemical Substances
- ICH Q 7 A:
  Good Manufacturing Practice for Active Pharmaceutical Ingredients

EU documents

- CPMP/QWP/130/96, Rev 1:
  Guideline on the Chemistry of New Active Substances
- CPMP/QWP/158/01 Rev:
  NfG on Quality of Water for Pharmaceutical Use
- CPMP/QWP/072/96:
  NfG on Start of Shelf-Life of the Finished Dosage Form
- CPMP/QWP/155/96:
  NfG on Development Pharmaceutics
- CPMP/QWP/054/98:
  Annex to NfG on Development Pharmaceutics (CPMP/QWP/155/96): Decision Trees for Selection of Sterilisation Methods.
- CPMP/QWP/130/96, Rev 1:
  Guideline on the Chemistry of New Active Substances

- CPMP/QWP/848/96:
  NfG on Process Validation
- CPMP/QWP/2054/03:
  Annex II to NfG on Process Validation:
  Non-Standard Processes
- CPMP/QWP/159/96:
  NfG on Maximum Shelf-Life for Sterile Products after First Opening or following Reconstitution
- CPMP/QWP/486/95:
  NfG on Manufacture of the Finished Dosage Form
- CPMP/QWP/419/03:
  NfG on Excipients, Antioxidants and Antimicrobial Preservatives in the Dossier for Application for Marketing Authorisation of a Medicinal Product
- CPMP/QWP/4539/03:
  Guideline on Plastic Primary Packaging Materials
- CPMP/QWP/297/97 Rev. 1:
  NfG on Summary of Requirements for Active Substances in Part II of the Dossier
- CPMP/SWP/QWP/4446/00:
  NfG on Specification Limits for Residues of Metal Catalysts
- EMEA/410/01 Rev. 2:
  NfG on Minimizing the Risk of Transmitting Animal Spongiform Encephalopathy Agents via Human and Veterinary Medicinal Products

FDA documents

- Container Closure Systems for Packaging Human Drugs and Biologics
- Environmental Assessment of Human Drug and Biologics Applications
- Format and Content of the Chemistry, Manufacturing and Controls Section of an Application
- INDs for Phase 2 and 3 Studies; Chemistry, Manufacturing, and Controls Information
- NDAs: Impurities in Drug Substances
- Submission Documentation for Sterilization Process Validation in Applications for Human and Veterinary Drug Products.
- Submission of Chemistry, Manufacturing and Controls Information for Synthetic Peptide Substances
- Submitting Documentation for the Manufacturing of and Controls for Drug Products
- Submitting Documentation for the Stability of Human Drugs and Biologics
- Submitting Samples and Analytical Data for Methods Validation
- Submitting Supporting Documentation in Drug Applications for the Manufacture of Drug Substances
- Submitting Supporting Documentation in Drug Applications for the Manufacture of Drug Products
- Drug Product: Chemistry, Manufacturing, and Controls Information (Draft)
- Drug Substance: Chemistry, Manufacturing, and Controls Information (Draft)

- Stability Testing of Drug Substances and Drug Products (Draft)
- Manufacture, Processing or Holding of Active Pharmaceutical Ingredients (Draft)
- Sterile Drug Products Produced by Aseptic Processing – Current Good Manufacturing Practice
- Preparation of Investigational New Drug Products (Human and Animal)

Non-clinical guidelines
ICH documents

- ICH M4 Safety:
  Nonclinical Summaries and Organisation of Module 4
- ICH M 3:
  Non-Clinical Safety Studies for the Conduct of Human Clinical Trials for Pharmaceuticals
- ICH S 1 A:
  Need for Long-term Rodent Carcinogenicity Studies of Pharmaceuticals
- ICH S 1 B:
  Testing for Carcinogenicity of Pharmaceuticals
- ICH S 1 C:
  Dose Selection for Carcinogenicity Study of Pharmaceuticals.
- ICH S 2 A:
  Genotoxicity: Guidance on Specific Aspects of Regulatory Genotoxicity Tests for Pharmaceuticals
- ICH S 2 B:
  Genotoxicity: A Standard Battery for Genotoxicity Testing of Pharmaceuticals
- ICH S 3 A:
  Toxicokinetics: A Guidance for Assessing Systemic Exposure in Toxicology Studies
- ICH S 3 B:
  Pharmacokinetics: Guidance for Repeated Dose Tissue Distribution Studies
- ICH S 4 A:
  Duration of Chronic Toxicity Testing in Animals
- ICH S 5 A:
  Reproductive Toxicology: Detection of Toxicity to Reproduction for Medicinal Products
- ICH S 5 B:
  Reproductive Toxicology: Toxicity on Male Fertility
- ICH S 7 A:
  Safety Pharmacology Studies for Human Pharmaceuticals
- ICH S 7 B:
  Safety Pharmacology Studies for assessing the potential for Delayed Ventricular Repolarization (QT Interval Prolongation) by Human Pharmaceuticals

EU documents

- CPMP/SWP/1042/99 corr.:
  NfG on Repeated Dose Toxicity
- CPMP/SWP/2145/00:
  NfG on Non-Clinical Local Tolerance Testing of Medicinal Products
- CPMP/986/96:
  PtC in the Assessment of the Potential for QT Interval Prolongation by Non-cardiovascular Medicinal Products
- CPMP/SWP/4447/00:
  NfG on Environmental Risk Assessment on Medicinal Products for Human Use
- CPMP/SWP/5199/02:
  Position Paper on the Limits of Genotoxic Impurities
- EudraLex 3BS11A:
  Note for Pharmacokinetics and metabolic studies in the safety evaluation of new medicinal products in animals
- EudraLex Vol. 3C
  Note for guidance on pharmacokinetic studies in man
- EudraLex 3CC29A
  Investigation of chiral active substances
- EudraLex Vol. 4
  Good manufacturing practices - Annex 13 (Manufacture of Investigational Medicinal Products)

FDA documents

- Carcinogenicity Study Protocol Submissions
- Format and Content of the Nonclinical Pharmacology/Toxicology Section of an Application
- Immunotoxicology Evaluation of Investigational New Drugs
- Photosafety Testing
- Single Dose Acute Toxicity Testing for Pharmaceuticals - Revised
- Integration of Study Results to Access Concerns About Human Reproductive and Developmental Toxicities
- Nonclinical Studies for Development of Pharmaceutical Excipients
- Statistical Aspects of the Design, Analysis, and Interpretation of Chronic Rodent Carcinogenicity Studies of Pharmaceuticals

Clinical guidelines

ICH documents

- ICH M4 Efficacy:
  Clinical Overview, Clinical Summary, Sample Tables for Clinical Summary and Module V
- ICH E 2 A:
  Good Clinical Safety Data Management: Definitions and Standards for Expedited Reporting
- ICH E 3:
  Structure and Content of Clinical Study Reports
- ICH E 4:
  Dose Response Information to support Drug Registration
- ICH E 6:
  Guideline for Good Clinical Practice
- ICH E 8:
  General Considerations for Clinical Trials
- ICH E 9:
  Statistical Principles for Clinical Trials
- ICH E 10:
  Choice of Control Group and Related Issues for Clinical Trials
- ICH E 14:
  The Clinical Evaluation of QT/QTs Interval Prolongation and Proarrhythmic Potential for Non-Antiarrhythmic drugs

EU documents

- CPMP/EWP/205/95 rev. 2 – corr.:
  NfG on Evaluation of Anticancer Medicinal Products in Man
- CPMP/EWP/569/02:
  NfG on Evaluation of Anticancer Medicinal Products in Man: Addendum on Pediatric Oncology
- CPMP/EWP/560/95
  NfG on the Investigation of Drug Interactions
- CPMP/EWP/908/99:
  PtC on Multiplicity Issues in Clinical Trials
- CPMP/EWP/2330/99:
  PtC on Application with 1.) Meta-analyses and 2.) One Pivotal study
- CPMP/EWP/2863/99:
  PtC on Adjustment for baseline Covariates
- CPMP/EWP/2747/00:
  NfG on Co-ordinating Investigator Signature of Clinical Study Reports
- CPMP/EWP/2998/03:
  NfG on the Inclusion of Appendices to Clinical Study Reports in Marketing Authorisation Applications

FDA documents
- Cancer Drug and Biological Products - Clinical Data in Marketing Applications
- Providing Clinical Evidence of Effectiveness for Human Drug and Biological Products
- Study and Evaluation of Gender Differences in the Clinical Evaluation of Drugs.
- Study of Drugs Likely to be used in the Elderly.
- Submission of Abbreviated Reports and Synopses in Support of Marketing Applications.
- Available Therapy
- Pediatric Oncology Studies in Response to a Written Request
- Premarketing Risk Assessment (Draft)
- Drug Metabolism/Drug Interaction Studies in the Drug Development Process: Studies In Vitro (Draft)
- In Vivo Metabolism/Drug Interaction Studies - Study Design, Data Analysis, and Recommendations for Dosing and Labeling
- Exposure-Response Relationships - Study Design, Data Analysis, and Regulatory Applications
- Information Program on Clinical Trials for Serious or Life-Threatening Diseases and Conditions
- Information Program on Clinical Trials for Serious or Life-Threatening Diseases: Establishment of a Data Bank
- Fast Track Drug Development Programs: Designation, Development, and Application Review
- Pharmacogenomic Data Submissions

APPENDIX 20 SUMMARY TABLE CONCERNING THE REGULATORY STRATEGY FOR THE MA FOR THE DIFFERENT COUNTRIES

Planned sending date	Planned submission date	Country	Area	Marketing Priority	Scenario	Master Dossier
Q1, 2011	Q1, 2011	EU	EU	1		M1
Q1, 2011	Q1, 2011	USA	USA	1		M1
Q1/Q2, 2011	Q1/Q2, 2011	Switzerland	CH	2		M1
Q1/Q2, 2011	Q1/Q2, 2011	Japan	JP	1		M1
Q3/2011		Australia	SEA	1	1	M1
Q3/2011		South Korea	SEA	1	1	M1
Q3/2011		Russia	EE	1	1	M1int
Q3/2011		South Africa		2	1	M1
Q2/2012		Lebanon	AF	1	2	M2 int.
Q2/2012		Belarus	EE	1	2	M2 int.
Q2/2012		Israel	EE	1	2	M2
Q2/2012		Kazakhstan	EE	1	2	M2 int.
Q2/2012		Turkey	EE	1	2	M2 int.
Q2/2012		Ukraine	EE	1	2	M2 int.
Q2/2012		Argentina	LA	1	2	M2 int.
Q2/2012		Chile	LA	1	2	M2 int.
Q2/2012		Colombia	LA	1	2	M2 int.
Q2/2012		Mexico	LA	1	2	M2 int.
Q2/2012		Venezuela	LA	1	2	M2 int.
Q2/2012		Iran	ME	1	2	M2 int.
Q2/2012		Kuwait	ME	1	2	M2 int.
Q2/2012		Saudi Arabia	ME	1	2	M2 int.
Q2/2012		UAE	ME	1	2	M2 int.
Q2/2012		China	SEA	1	2	M2 int.
Q2/2012		India	SEA	1	2	M2 int.
Q2/2012		Singapore	SEA	1	2	M2 int.
Q2/2012		Taiwan	SEA	1	2	M2 int.
Q3,2012		Algeria	AF	2	2	M2 int.
Q3,2012		Morocco	AF	2	2	M2 int.
Q3,2012		Croatia	EE	2	2	M2 int.
Q3,2012		Montenegro	EE	2	2	M2 int.
Q3,2012		Serbia	EE	2	2	M2 int.
Q3,2012		Brazil	LA	2	2	M2 int.
Q3,2012		Costa Rica	LA	2	2	M2 int.
Q3,2012		Dom. Rep.	LA	2	2	M2 int.
Q3,2012		Ecuador	LA	2	2	M2 int.
Q3,2012		El Salvador	LA	2	2	M2 int.
Q3,2012		Guatemala	LA	2	2	M2 int.
Q3,2012		Honduras	LA	2	2	M2 int.
Q3,2012		Nicaragua	LA	2	2	M2 int.
Q3,2012		Panama	LA	2	2	M2 int.

Planned sending date	Planned submission date	Country	Area	Marketing Priority	Scenario	Master Dossier
Q3,2012		Peru	LA	2	2	M2 int.
Q3,2012		Uruguay	LA	2	2	M2 int.
Q3,2012		Bahrain	ME	2	2	M2 int.
Q3,2012		Egypt	ME	2	2	M2 int.
Q3,2012		Oman	ME	2	2	M2 int.
Q3,2012		Qatar	ME	2	2	M2 int.
Q3,2012		Hong Kong	SEA	2	2	M2 int.
Q3,2012		Indonesia	SEA	2	2	M2 int.
Q3,2012		Malaysia	SEA	2	2	M2 int.
Q3,2012		New Zealand	SEA	2	2	M2 int.
Q3,2012		Philippines	SEA	2	2	M2 int.
Q3,2012		Thailand	SEA	2	2	M2 int.
Q3,2012		Vietnam	SEA	2	2	M2 int.

APPENDIX 21 REQUIREMENTS TABLES

Approval Time (months)	12	18-24		12-18
Comments				
Regulatory procedure e.g. fast track, orphan drug, priority review			abridged evaluation within 2 months	
Other documents			two assessment reports of two benchmarking	
Plan master file				
Price certificate				
Declaration for cold chain				
Trademark certificate				
Power of attorney to register, market and disribute (notarized?)				
Supply agreement				
GMP legalized (notarized and legalized)		yes	yes	yes
No. of Samples		?	2	1
Samples demonstration/analysis		analysis	demonstration	
Regulatory status list	yes	yes	yes	yes
Translations	no	yes	no	no
Mock-ups	yes	yes	yes	yes
Labeling	yes	yes	yes	yes
PI	yes	yes	yes	yes
SPC US/EU	US/EU	US/EU	US/EU	US/EU
Module 5	yes	yes	no	yes
Module 4	yes	yes	no	yes
Module 3 abbr.	no	yes	yes	yes
Module 3 full	yes	no	no	no
Module 2	yes	yes	yes	yes
CPP EU	no	yes	yes	no
CPP US	no	yes	no	yes
Country	Australia	China	Singapore	Taiwan

		Croatia	Turkey
Approval Time (months)		15	24-36
Regulatory procedure e.g. fast track, orphan drug, priority review		priority review	normal
Other documents			Public price of origin country, all registered country public price
Plan master file			yes
Price certificate		yes	yes
Declaration for cold chain		yes	yes
Trademark certificate		no	no
Power of attorney to register, market and disribute (notarized?)		no	yes
Supply agreement		no	no
GMP legalized (notarized and legalized)		yes	yes
No. of Samples		5	1**
Samples demonstration/analysis		analysis	demonstration
Regulatory status list		yes	yes
Translations		no	Module 2 and 3
Mock-ups		yes	yes
Labeling		yes	yes
PI		yes	yes
SPC US/EU		EU	US/EU
Clinical data			Phase III data mandatorily needed
Module 5		yes	yes
Module 4		yes	yes
Module 3 abbr.		yes	yes
Module 2		yes	yes
CPP EU		yes	yes*
CPP US			yes
Country		Croatia	Turkey

Approval Time (months)	12	10
Regulatory procedure e.g. fast track, orphan drug, priority review		
Other documents	1. inspection of manufacturer may be required; 2. Batch records of three batches; 3 flow chart of the manufacturing; 4. Site master file; 5 - original PIL	Stability study signed by the head of quality assurance; Certificate of Analysis of one batch of DS and three batches of DP incl. Chromatograms, batch records
Plan master file	yes	
Price certificate		
Declaration for cold chain	yes	
Trademark certificate	yes	yes
Power of attorney to register, market and disribute (notarized?)	yes	yes
Supply agreement		
GMP legalized (notarized and legalized)	necessary	yes
No. of samples	1	1
Samples demonstration/analysis	demonstration	analysis
Regulatory status list	yes	
Translations	yes	yes
Mock-ups	yes	yes
Labeling	yes	yes
PI	yes	yes
SPC US/EU	US/EU	US/EU
Clinical data	Phase III data mandatorily needed	Published clinical literature
Module 5	no	no
Module 4	no	no
Module 3 abbr.	yes	yes
Module 3 full	no	no
Module 2	yes	yes
CPP EU	yes	yes
CPP US	yes	yes
Country	Brazil	Mexico

Approval Time (months)	15		24-36
Regulatory procedure e.g. fast track, orphan drug, priority review	priority review		normal
Other documents	Original EU dossier plus CHMP opinion, Commission decision, EU Assessment Reports, AtOs during the EU procedure, statements		Public price of origin country, all registered country public price and their VAT rate, FOB price and DMF for the compound
Plan master file	""		yes
Price certificate	yes		yes
Declaration for cold chain	yes		yes
Trademark certificate	no		no
Power of attorney to register, market and disribute (notarized?)	no		yes
Supply agreement	no		no
GMP legalized (notarized and legalized)	yes		yes
No. of Samples	5		1**
Samples demonstration/analysis	analysis		demonstration
Regulatory status list	yes		""
Translations	no		Module 2 and 3
Mock-ups	yes		yes
Labeling	yes		yes
PI	yes		yes
SPC US/EU	EU		US/EU
Clinical data	""		Phase III data mandatorily needed
Module 5	yes		yes
Module 4	yes		yes
Module 3 abbr.	no		yes
Module 3 full	yes		no
Module 2	yes		yes
CPP EU	yes		yes*
CPP US	""		yes
Country	Croatia		Turkey

Approval Time (months)	12	10
Regulatory procedure e.g. fast track, orphan drug, priority review		
Other documents	1. inspection of manufacturer may be required; 2. Batch records of three batches; 3 flow chart of the manufacturing; 4. Site master file; 5 - original PIL	Stability study signed by the head of quality assurance, Certificate of Analysis of one batch of DS and three batches of DP incl. Chromatograms, batch records
Plan master file	yes	
Price certificate		
Declaration for cold chain	yes	
Trademark certificate	yes	yes
Power of attorney to register, market and disribute (notarized?)	yes	yes
Supply agreement		
GMP legalized (notarized and legalized)	yes	yes
No. of Samples	1	1
Samples demonstration/analysis	demonstration	analysis
Regulatory status list	yes	
Translations	yes	yes
Mock-ups	yes	yes
Labeling	yes	yes
PI	yes	yes
SPC US/EU	US/EU	US/EU
Clinical data	Phase III data mandatorily needed	Published clinical literature
Module 5	no	no
Module 4	no	no
Module 3 abbr.	yes	yes
Module 3 full	no	no
Module 2	yes	yes
CPP EU	yes	yes
CPP US	yes	yes
Country	Brazil	Mexico

Approval Time (months)	12	18-24
Regulatory procedure e.g. fast track, orphan drug, priority review		
Other documents		
Plan master file		
Price certificate		
Declaration for cold chain		
Trademark certificate		
Power of attorney to register, market and disribute (notarized?)		
Supply agreement		
GMP legalized (notarized and legalized)		yes
No. of Samples		?
Samples demonstration/analysis		analysis
Regulatory status list	yes	yes
Translations	no	yes
Mock-ups	yes	yes
Labeling	yes	yes
PI	yes	yes
SPC US/EU	US/EU	US/EU
Clinical data		
Module 5	yes	yes
Module 4	yes	yes
Module 3 abbr.	no	yes
Module 3 full	yes	no
Module 2	yes	yes
CPP EU	no	yes
CPP US	no	yes
Country	Australia	China

Approval Time (months)		12-18
Regulatory procedure e.g. fast track, orphan drug, priority review	abridged evaluation within 2 months	
Other documents	two assessment reports of two benchmarking Authorities e.g. EMA and FDA	
Plan master file		
Price certificate		
Declaration for cold chain		
Trademark certificate		
Power of attorney to register, market and disribute (notarized?)		
Supply agreement		
GMP legalized (notarized and legalized)	yes	yes
No. of Samples	2	1
Samples demonstration/analysis	demonstration	
Regulatory status list		
Translations	no	no
Mock-ups	yes	yes
Labeling	yes	yes
PI	yes	yes
SPC US/EU	US/EU	US/EU
Clinical data		
Module 5	yes	yes
Module 4	yes	yes
Module 3 abbr.	yes	yes
Module 3 full	no	no
Module 2	yes	yes
CPP EU	yes	no
CPP US	no	yes
Country	Singapore	Taiwan

9   Bibliography

1. Official Journal L 214, 24.08.1993 - Council Regulation (EEC) No 2309/93 of 22 July 1993 laying down Community procedures for the authorisation and supervision of medicinal products for human and veterinary use and establishing a European Agency for the Evaluation of Medicinal Products – page 1 - 21

   http://ec.europa.eu/enterprise/pharmaceuticals/eudralex/vol1_en.htm - dated 27.04.2009

   (Official Journal L 214, 24/8/1993 p. 1 - 21; Finnish special edition: Chapter 13 Volume 24 p. 158; Swedish special edition: Chapter 13 Volume 24 p. 158).

   http://www.fve.org/veterinary/pdf/medicines/regulation_2309_93_en.pdf

2. Official Journal L 136, 30.04.2004 - Regulation (EC) No 726/2004 of the European Parliament and of the Council of 31 March 2004 laying down Community procedures for the authorisation and supervision of medicinal products for human and veterinary use and establishing a European Medicines Agency – page 1 ff.

   (OJ L 136, 30.4.2004, p. 1)

   http://ec.europa.eu/health/files/eudralex/vol-1/reg_2004_726_cons/reg_2004_726_cons_en.pdf - dated 27.04.2009

3. Official Journal L 311, 28.11.2001 - Directive 2001/83/EEC of the European Parliament and of the Council of 6 November 2001 on the Community code relating to medicinal products for human use – page 67 - 128

   http://eudravigilance.emea.europa.eu/human/docs/Directives/Consolidated2001-83EN.pdf – dated 27.04.2009

   Official Journal L – 311, 28/11/2004, p. 67 – 128

   http://ec.europa.eu/enterprise/pharmaceuticals/eudralex/vol1_en.htm – dated 27.04.2009

   DIRECTIVE 2001/83/EC OF THE EUROPEAN PARLIAMENT AND OF THE COUNCIL

   of 6 November 2001 on the Community code relating to medicinal products for human use

   (OJ L 311, 28.11.2001, p. 67)

4. Official Journal L 136, 30.04.2004 - Directive 2004/27 EEC of the European Parliament and of the Council of 31 March 2004 amending Directive 2001/83/EC on the Community code relating to medicinal products for human use – page 34 - 57

   (Official Journal L 136, 30/4/2004 p. 34 - 57).

   http://ec.europa.eu/health/files/eudralex/vol-1/dir_2004_27/dir_2004_27_en.pdf - dated 27.04.2009

5. Official Journal L 136, 30.04.2004 - Directive 2004/24/EC of the European Parliament and of the Council of 31 March 2004 amending, as regards traditional herbal medicinal products, Directive 2001/83/EC on the Community code relating to medicinal products for human use – page 85 - 90

   (Official Journal L 136, 30/4/2004, p. 85 - 90).

   http://ec.europa.eu/enterprise/pharmaceuticals/eudralex/vol-1/dir_2004_24/dir_2004_24_en.pdf - dated 27.04.2009

   http://eur-lex.europa.eu/LexUriServ/LexUriServ.do?uri=OJ:L:2004:136:0085:0090:en:PDF

6. Procedure on the granting of marketing authorisations by CADREAC Drug Regulatory Authorities for medicinal products for human use already authorized in the EU following the centralized procedure and the variation and renewal of such marketing authorisations (5th revision of December 21,2001)

7. Procedure on the granting of marketing authorisations by CADREAC Drug Regulatory Authorities for medicinal products for human use already authorized in EU member states following the decentralized procedure (1st revision of June 10,2010)

8. Homepage of ASEAN (Association of Southeast Asian Nationals http://www.aseansec.org - dated 27.04.2009

9. Homepage of ICH (International Conference of Harmonization:

    The Fifth International Conference on Harmonization - ICH5 and Steering Committee Meeting

    "The Common Technical Document Released Putting It All Together A Decade of Harmonization"

    http://www.ich.org/cache/html/454-272-1.html - dated 27.04.2009

10. Volume 2B NtA: Medicinal products for human use - Presentation and format of the dossier Common Technical Document (CTD)

    http://ec.europa.eu/enterprise/pharmaceuticals/eudralex/vol2_en.htm#2b

    http://ec.europa.eu/enterprise/pharmaceuticals/eudralex/vol-2/b/update_200805/ctd_05-2008.pdf - dated 27.04.2009

11. http://en.wikipedia.org/wiki/File:CTD_Pyramid.jpg

12. VOLUME 2A NtA - Procedures for marketing authorisation CHAPTER 1 Marketing authorisation from November 2005

    http://ec.europa.eu/enterprise/pharmaceuticals/eudralex/vol-2/a/vol2a_chap1_2005-11.pdf - dated 27.04.2009

13. Guideline on the procedure for accelerated assessment pursuant to articile 14(9) of regulation (EC) No 726/2004

    http://www.emea.europa.eu/docs/en_GB/document_library/Regulatory_and_procedural_guideline/2009/10/WC500004136.pdf - dated 27.04.2009

14. EMA Website (http://www.emea.eu.int/ – Human Medicines - Application procedures - 'Pre-Submission Guidance' - dated 27.04.2009

    http://www.ema.europa.eu/ema/index.jsp?curl=pages/regulation/general/general_content_000119.jsp&murl=menus/regulations/regulations.jsp&mid=WC0b01ac0580022974 - dated 27.08.2010

15. VOLUME 2A NtA - Procedures for marketing authorisation - CHAPTER 4 - Centralized Procedure from April 2006

    http://ec.europa.eu/enterprise/pharmaceuticals/eudralex/vol-2/a/chap4rev200604%20.pdf

    dated 21.07.2009

16. VOLUME 2A Notice to applicants - Procedures for marketing authorisation - CHAPTER 2 - Mutual Recognition from February 2007

    http://ec.europa.eu/enterprise/pharmaceuticals/eudralex/vol-2/a/vol2a_chap2_2007-02.pdf

    Dated 22.07.2009

17. Best practice guide for decentralised and mutual recognition procedures, October 1996, revision May 2007 (CMD – Coordination group for mutual recognition procedures and decentralized procedures – human)

    http://www.hma.eu/fileadmin/dateien/Human_Medicines/CMD_h_/procedural_guidance/Application_for_MA/BPG_MRP_DCP_2007_05_Rev6_Clean.pdf

18. http://www.fda.gov/

19. Federal Register Vol. 68, No. 72, April 15, 2003 – Draft Guidance - Guidance for Industry-submitting MAs according to the ICH CTD format
    http://edocket.access.gpo.gov/2003/pdf/03-8802.pdf
    18248 - Federal Register / Vol. 68, No. 72 / Tuesday, April 15, 2003 / Notices
20. Form FDA-356h "Application to market a new drug, biologic or an antibiotic drug for human use" (Title 21, Code of Federal Regulations parts 314 and 610)
    http://www.fda.gov/opacom/morechoices/fdaforms/internal/FDA-356h.pdf
21. Code of Federal Regulations, Title 21 – Foods and Drugs, Volume 5, Revised as of April 1, 2008 (CITE: 21 CFR 314.50)
    Chapter 1 – Food and drugs administration department of health and human services
    Subchapter D – drugs for human use
    Part 314 – Applications for FDA approval to market a new drug
    Subpart B – Applications
    Section 314.50 – Content and format of an application
    http://www.accessdata.fda.gov/scripts/cdrh/cfdocs/cfcfr/CFRSearch.cfm?CFRPart=314
    http://www.accessdata.fda.gov/scripts/cdrh/cfdocs/cfcfr/CFRSearch.cfm?fr=314.50
22. Code of Federal Regulations, Title 21 – 21 CFR Part 314.110 effective August 11, 2008
    http://edocket.access.gpo.gov/2008/pdf/E8-15610.pdf and
    http://law.justia.com/us/cfr/title21/21-5.0.1.1.4.4.1.10.html dated 01.09.2009
23. Freedom of Information (FOI) Act per 21 CFR Part 20 (cf. XXX)
    http://www.fda.gov/AboutFDA/ReportsManualsForms/StaffManualGuides/ucm138408.htm - dated 01.09.2009
24. Susan Thaul, FDA Fast Track and Priority Review Programs, CRS Report of Congress - Order Code RS22814, February 21, 2008
    http://www.nationalaglawcenter.org/assets/crs/RS22814.pdf - dated 01.09.2009
25. Food and Drug Administration Modernization Act of 1997 (FDAMA, P.L. 105-115)
    http://www.fda.gov/RegulatoryInformation/Legislation/FederalFoodDrugandCosmeticActFDCAct/SignificantAmendmentstotheFDCAct/FDAMA/FullTextofFDAMAlaw/default.htm - dated 22.10.2009
26. http://www.dgra.de/studiengang/pdf/master_hoerner_a.pdf - dated 22.10.2009
27. CADREAC SOP: CADREAC SOP-3 (2001) - Responsibilities and function of CADREAC secretariat
    http://old.sukl.cz/en06/en0601.htm - dated 27.04.2009
28. CADREAC homepage -
    http://web.archive.org/web/20040605093650/http://www.cadreac.org - dated 27.04.2009
29. Common CADREAC Procedure (CCP) for retrospective inclusion of centrally authorized medicinal products for human use in the Common CADREAC Simplified System - in force since May 2001 http://www.milray.org/pdf/CADREAC.pdf - dated 27.04.2009
30. http://www.newcadreac.org/members.html- dated 27.04.2009
31. Procedure on the granting of marketing authorisations by new CADREAC (nCADREAC) Drug Regulatory Authorities for medicinal products for human use already authorised in the EU member states following the centralized procedure and the variation and renewal of such marketing authorisations
    http://www.newcadreac.org/simp_procedures.html - dated 27.04.2009

32. Procedure on the granting of marketing authorisations by new CADREAC (nCADREAC) Drug Regulatory Authorities for medicinal products for human use already authorised in EU member states following the mutual recognition procedure and the variation and renewal of such marketing authorisations

    http://www.newcadreac.org/simp_procedures.html - dated 27.04.2009

33. The ASEAN Common Technical Document (ACTD) for the registration of pharmaceuticals for human use – organization of the dossier

    http://www.hsa.gov.sg/publish/etc/medialib/hsa_library/health_products_regulation/western_medicines/files_guidelines.Par.22449.File.dat/ACTD_OrganizationofDossier.pdf

34. http://upload.wikimedia.org/wikipedia/en/a/a9/CTD_Pyramid.jpg - dated 27.04.2009

    http://www.ectdblog.com/2008_05_01_archive.html

35. http://1.bp.blogspot.com/_Yjwi3JtqDOY/SERNIifkrEI/AAAAAAAAKsQ/Zr22lcsU1R8/s1600-h/actd.png - dated 27.04.2009

    http://www.ectdblog.com/2008_05_01_archive.html

36. The ASEAN Common Technical Dossier (ACTD) for the registration of pharmaceuticals for human use – Part II Quality

    http://www.hsa.gov.sg/publish/etc/medialib/hsa_library/health_products_regulation/western_medicines/files_guidelines.Par.28201.File.dat/ACTD_PartIIQuality_Apr05.pdf

    http://www.hsa.gov.sg/publish/hsaportal/en/health_products_regulation/western_medicines/guidelines.html

37. The ASEAN Common Technical Dossier (ACTD) for the registration of pharmaceuticals for human use – Part III Nonclinical document

    http://www.hsa.gov.sg/publish/hsaportal/en/health_products_regulation/western_medicines/guidelines.html

    http://www.hsa.gov.sg/publish/etc/medialib/hsa_library/health_products_regulation/western_medicines/files_guidelines.Par.59468.File.dat/ACTD_PartIIINonClinical_Nov05.pdf

38. The ASEAN Common Technical Dossier (ACTD) for the registration of pharmaceuticals for human use – Part IV Clinical document

    http://www.hsa.gov.sg/publish/hsaportal/en/health_products_regulation/western_medicines/guidelines.html

    http://www.hsa.gov.sg/publish/etc/medialib/hsa_library/health_products_regulation/western_medicines/files_guidelines.Par.54671.File.dat/ACTD_PartIVClinical_Nov05.pdf

39. Guidance on Medicinal Product Registration in Singapore (effective January 1, 2009)

    http://www.hsa.gov.sg/publish/hsaportal/en/health_products_regulation/western_medicines/guidelines.html

    http://www.hsa.gov.sg/publish/etc/medialib/hsa_library/health_products_regulation/western_medicines/files_guidelines.Par.15295.File.dat/Guidance%20on%20Medicinal%20Product%20Registration%20in%20Singapore%202009_Complete%20with%20Appendices.pdf

40. Homepage of Health Sciences Authority – health products regulations - medicines: http://www.hsa.gov.sg/publish/hsaportal/en/health_products_regulation/western_medicines.html - dated 27.04.2009

41. Drug Registration Regulation (SFDA Order 28) (Translation by RDPAC, for Member use only)

    Drug Registration Regulation was approved on June 18, 2007 by SFDA executive meeting and is hereby published, which become effective from October 1, 2007.

    SFDA Commissioner, Shao Minli, July 10, 2007

42. Annex 2: Registration Categories and Application Information Requirements of Chemical Drugs

43. Annex 3: Registration Categories and Application Information Items Requirements of Biological Products
44. Resolution RDC 315 of 26-Oct-2005 - Brazilian Official Gazette of 10/31/05
45. Resolution RDC 47 – 2009 of 08 September 2009 - Novas Regras para Bulas de Medicamentos
46. RESOLUTION - RDC N° 136 OF MAY 29, 2003 - UNION OFFICIAL GAZETTE OF 02/06/2003
47. Law 9.787 of 10-Feb-1999 - Brasília, February 10th 1999, 178th of the Independence and 111st of the Republic - FERNANDO HENRIQUE CARDOSO; José Serra

   http://www.anvisa.gov.br/hotsite/genericos/legis/leis/9787_e.htm - dated 22.07.2009
48. Decree 3.961 of 10-Oct-2001

49. http://www.anvisa.gov.br- dated 22.07.2009

50. Private information from Susan Koepke, Regulatory Affairs Director – Latin America, Merck Serono

51. Resolution RDC 314 of 09-Dec-2004)

52. Law n° 6.360, of September 23, 1976 -
OFFICIAL JOURNAL OF THE UNION OF SEPTEMBER 24, 1976 - Brasilia, September 23, 1976; 155 of Independence and 88 of the Republic. - Ernesto Geisel, Paulo de Almeida Machado

    http://www.anvisa.gov.br/hotsite/genericos/legis/leis/6360_e.htm- dated 22.07.2009
53. Resolution RDC 28 of 04.04.2007 - RESOLUÇÃO RDC No- 28, DE 4 DE ABRIL DE 2007 - Dispõe sobre a priorização da análise técnica de petições, no âmbito da Gerência- Geral de Medicamentos da ANVISA, cuja relevância pública se enquadre nos termos desta Resolução. - DIRCEU RAPOSO DE MELLO
54. Resolution RDC 16 of 13.03.2008 - RESOLUÇÃO N° 16, DE 13 DE MARÇO DE 2008

    Altera a Resolução - RDC n° 28, de 4 de abril de 2007, que dispõe sobre a priorização de análise técnica de petições no âmbito da Gerência Geral de Medicamentos da ANVISA - DIRCEU RAPOSO DE MELLO
55. Decree 5775/2006 - DECRETO No- 5.775, DE 10 DE MAIO DE 2006

    Dispõe sobre o fracionamento de medicamentos, dá nova redação aos arts. 2o e 9o

    do Decreto no 74.170, de 10 de junho de 1974, e dá outras providências - Brasília, 10 de maio de 2006; 185o da Independência e 118o da República - LUIZ INÁCIO LULA DA SILVA, José Agenor Álvares da Silva
56. http://www.anvisa.gov.br/servicos/consulta_documentos.htm - dated 22.07.2009

57. http://en.wikipedia.org/wiki/Monoclonal_antibodies - dated 10.05.2010

58. http://upload.wikimedia.org/wikipedia/commons/9/9a/Monoclonals.png - dated 10.05.2010

59. http://en.wikipedia.org/wiki/Epidermal_growth_factor_receptor

60. http://en.wikipedia.org/wiki/Biomarker - dated 25.08.2010

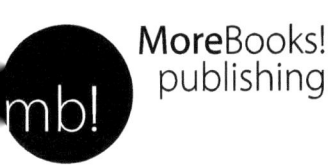
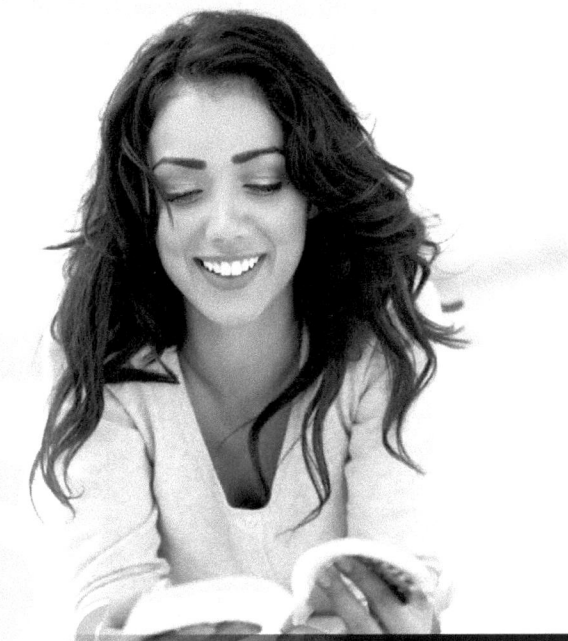

i want morebooks!

Buy your books fast and straightforward online - at one of world's fastest growing online book stores! Environmentally sound due to Print-on-Demand technologies.

Buy your books online at
www.get-morebooks.com

Kaufen Sie Ihre Bücher schnell und unkompliziert online – auf einer der am schnellsten wachsenden Buchhandelsplattformen weltweit! Dank Print-On-Demand umwelt- und ressourcenschonend produziert.

Bücher schneller online kaufen
www.morebooks.de

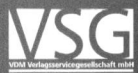

VDM Verlagsservicegesellschaft mbH
Heinrich-Böcking-Str. 6-8   Telefon: +49 681 3720 174   info@vdm-vsg.de
D - 66121 Saarbrücken   Telefax: +49 681 3720 1749   www.vdm-vsg.de

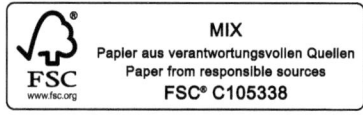

Printed by Books on Demand GmbH, Norderstedt / Germany